Advance Praise for
Intermittent Fasting Transformation

"Women shouldn't intermittent fast like men! Whether you are cycling, in perimenopause, or menopause, Cynthia's IF45 plan will fit your needs to boost energy levels, improve sleep quality, prevent weight gain, and feel better than ever in your body."

—JJ Virgin, *New York Times* bestselling author of *The Virgin Diet*

"Intermittent fasting will change how you feel every single day. It will keep you young or even reverse the clock. Fasting is different for women. Read this book now to discover Cynthia Thurlow's unique take on fasting."

—Dave Asprey, author of *The Bulletproof Diet*

"Ever since Cynthia Thurlow's TEDx Talk, 'Intermittent Fasting: Transformational Technique,' went viral in 2019, she has been considered a top thought leader in the field of IF and women's health. Her new book, *Intermittent Fasting Transformation*, puts all of her best advice for women in one place. Spoiler alert: Intermittent fasting is safe for women, and Cynthia explains it through the lens of her personal journey and also her expertise as a nurse practitioner."

—Gin Stephens, *New York Times* bestselling author of *Fast. Feast. Repeat.*; *Clean(ish)*; and *Delay, Don't Deny*

"Fascinating and so accessible . . . Cynthia Thurlow has cracked the code on how hormones affect weight loss and why intermittent fasting is such a game-changer for women. It's a must-read for women looking for a nutrition plan that fits easily into their lives and takes their health and total wellness to the next level."

—Robb Wolf, bestselling author of *The Paleo Solution* and *Wired to Eat*

"This book is the complete guide to women's health. Cynthia outlines a brilliant 45-day program to harness the healing benefits of fasting. It's important to understand that women should practice intermittent fasting differently than men, and Cynthia shares how women of all ages can use this tool properly. This book will change the lives of so many!"

—Ben Azadi, bestselling author of *Keto Flex* and founder of Keto Kamp

"We have come to a point in time when well-designed programs to help optimize women is deeply needed in the face of an epidemic of confusion. We need Cynthia's work now more than ever. Her dedication to helping transform lives and commitment to good science practices is exceptional. She does a wonderful job in providing a framework for women to gain control of their health and weight. As a fellowship trained physician in the area of nutrition/obesity medicine and geriatrics as well as founder of The Institute for Muscle-Centric Medicine, I love Cynthia's work and am excited for it to get into the hands of the reader."

—Dr. Gabrielle Lyon, DO, founder of the
Institute for Muscle-Centric Medicine

"This groundbreaking, deeply researched book is the only diet plan truly tailored to women. But the benefits go far beyond weight loss—with Cynthia's plan, women can unlock their metabolic health to help slow down the effects of aging; protect themselves against disease; and feel energized, strong, and vibrant."

—Benjamin Bikman, PhD, scientist and author of *Why We Get Sick*

INTERMITTENT
FASTING
TRANSFORMATION

The 45-Day Program for Women to Lose Stubborn
Weight, Improve Hormonal Health, and Slow Aging

Cynthia Thurlow, NP

AVERY
an imprint of Penguin Random House
New York

AVERY

an imprint of Penguin Random House LLC
penguinrandomhouse.com

Most Avery books are available at special quantity discounts for bulk purchase for sales promotions, premiums, fund-raising, and educational needs. Special books or book excerpts also can be created to fit specific needs.
For details, write SpecialMarkets@penguinrandomhouse.com.

Library of Congress Cataloging-in-Publication Data

Names: Thurlow, Cynthia, author.
Title: Intermittent Fasting Transformation: the 45-day program for women to lose stubborn weight, improve hormonal health, and slow aging / by Cynthia Thurlow.
Description: New York: Avery, an imprint of Penguin Random House, [2022] | Includes index.
Identifiers: LCCN 2021056265 (print) | LCCN 2021056266 (ebook) | ISBN 9780593419311 (trade paperback) | ISBN 9780593419328 (epub)
Subjects: LCSH: Fasting. | Weight loss. | Women—Health and hygiene. | Fasting—Health aspects.
Classification: LCC RM226 .T48 2022 (print) | LCC RM226 (ebook) |
DDC 613.2/5—dc23/eng/20211117
LC record available at https://lccn.loc.gov/2021056265
LC ebook record available at https://lccn.loc.gov/2021056266

Printed in the United States of America
2nd Printing

Book design by Patrice Sheridan

To my loves . . . Todd (aka the hubs), my boys (Jack and Liam), and the "doods" (Cooper and Baxter); thank you for inspiring me to grow and stretch far beyond my wildest dreams

Contents

Part Three
Forty-five Days to Transformation
149

Introduction

As women, we all want a life filled with joy, vitality, and meaning, and there's nothing to say we can't have it. Our life expectancy is at an all-time high. Our health habits are at an all-time high, too. We're eating better, exercising smarter but not harder, and learning how to find balance in our much fuller lives. We have everything going for us and there's so much to look forward to. But as we get older, we notice we're no longer as energetic or as young as we used to be. We just don't feel like ourselves.

Have you ever felt this way? If so, I'd like to introduce you to someone.

She worked a demanding job as a nurse practitioner. It was intellectually rigorous, with long hours of attending to the demands of her patients, their families, and other colleagues.

On top of that, she had two boys in elementary school and felt like her schedule had forced her to miss out on much of what was going on in their lives. She couldn't sleep through the night. In the morning, she had barely enough energy to drag herself out of bed. She was gaining weight and felt fat and frumpy.

Filled with frustration, she continued this go-go-go existence. She tried to improve her symptoms with changing her nutrition and diet but overdid it with too few carbs and too much exercise. Both made things worse.

She then suffered a severe gut infection and developed debilitating sensitivities to gluten and dairy. Her thyroid gland, responsible for metabolism and other functions, could not keep up. Instead of just enough cortisol—a stress hormone—to keep her alert and awake, with occasional extras for a fight-or-flight emergency, it stayed chronically elevated.

Hormonally, she was in the beginning stages of perimenopause—the five to seven years that precede menopause—and a time of wildly fluctuating hormones. Her progesterone was dropping, and her estrogen was up and down. These hormonal swings worsened her weight gain and created unrelenting food cravings. The stressors in her life only added to her hormonal upheaval.

Enough was enough. She decided to change her lifestyle. She stopped overexercising, switched to a gentler activity like yoga, removed inflammatory foods from her diet, and stopped under-nourishing her body. Yet her weight would not budge. Not a single pound.

She finally acquiesced to going on prescription medication for her underactive thyroid. She believed that the extra pounds would magically drop off by taking the drug. They did not. Her well-meaning physician, family, and friends dismissed the weight gain and other symptoms with, "You're in your forties now. Get used to it. This is your new normal."

She was discouraged, wiped out, unsure of where to turn, and generally down about her failing health.

This woman was me. The cumulative impact of too much stress, too little sleep, and too few carbohydrates in my diet, combined with being a wife, mom, and busy clinician took its toll. My lifestyle no longer agreed with me. Clearly, I needed help.

Eventually, I found a simple and straightforward solution that changed everything: intermittent fasting. To my amazement, I discovered it healed my body, brought my hormones back into harmony, and made me feel amazing and in command of my life again. And I got healthy to lose weight.

So—what exactly is this miracle called intermittent fasting? You'll learn all about it in this book, but in simple terms, intermittent fasting is a strategy in which you eat less often, putting the emphasis on *when* you eat rather than *what* you eat.

At first, I was skeptical. Intermittent fasting seemed so radical, and so against conventional wisdom. After all, aren't we supposed to eat three healthy meals a day, with nutritious snacks in between?

The answer to that question, backed by a surprising amount of clinical proof, is: "not really." As I dug into the science, I learned about some amazing benefits of intermittent fasting. It restores our intrinsic rhythms, burns fat, regenerates our health right down to the cellular level, and stabilizes our hormones. In turn, we are less likely to develop obesity, diabetes, vascular diseases, and autoimmune disorders. We prevent "metabolic inflexibility," too—a term you'll hear me use often. If you're not metabolically flexible, you'll have a hard time efficiently using fats or carbohydrates for energy, and this can set you up for metabolic diseases like insulin resistance, high blood pressure, inflammation, and other conditions.

I was excited about what I had learned. And I knew I had to do something differently, since I was in such bad shape and not getting the results I wanted. So I decided to test intermittent fasting on a population of one— me (the proverbial N of 1).

The results were nothing short of transformative. I finally lost that weight. I balanced my crazy, out-of-whack hormones. I was more energetic and more focused with laser-beam mental clarity. I got more done in the morning because I was not eating or digesting food. Not only that, I was more productive throughout the day because my schedule no longer revolved around planning meals and snacks. Intermittent fasting changed my life—and I knew it would change the lives of the thousands of women I now work with. All of this led me to develop my IF:45 plan.

This unique plan takes an individualized approach to intermittent fasting that is designed expressly for women. We have our own unique anatomy (our structure) and physiology (function) that are not like men's. All of this involves hormones, which are different from day to day and vary significantly depending on our life stage—premenopausal, perimenopausal, menopausal, and afterward. There is no one-size-fits-all strategy to intermittent fasting—which makes IF:45 so different from other dietary regimens.

My Mission

With my IF:45 plan, I'm helping women look and feel better than they could ever imagine—which is my major professional and career focus. Getting to this point in my career, however, involved lots of twists and turns along the way.

For background, I'm a nurse practitioner—that's a registered nurse with a graduate degree in adult primary care. We evaluate patients, make diagnoses, and admit them to hospitals. We prescribe medications and provide treatments, like physicians do. There has been a boom in this field that no one could have foreseen back in the 1990s, and today many people are putting their health care into our hands.

I did not set out to pursue a career in medicine. I began as a prelaw student with the goal of becoming an attorney. Although I got great grades and I loved to study the law, I did not want to practice it, so I did not pursue that path. Instead, I went to work for a computer company, but I was miserable. Life wasn't—and isn't—meant to be lived that way.

What pivoted me into health care was my dog. I had always wanted a dog and was finally able to own one. Caring for my beloved pet and her health made me realize how much I loved tending to the well-being of all creatures—both human and animals. That's when I decided to go back to school to take premed classes. It is ironic how a pet can change your life.

It turned out that premed was yet another detour on my career path, though. A professor of mine said, "Don't go to med school. You'll be miserable. Become a nurse practitioner instead."

The advice sank in and made sense. After all, I came from a long line of nurses and physicians. It was the family business. I finally realized it was my calling, and so the trajectory of my career changed, this time for good.

I finally had a clear vision for myself. I knew I was worthy and capable—and could make a difference in health care. I eventually obtained both my undergraduate and graduate degrees from Johns Hopkins University. Initially, I chose Hopkins because I had developed a deep interest in HIV and AIDS research and worked as a student intern on their prestigious HIV floor.

The work was fulfilling but a little slow-paced. I'm a total adrenaline junkie and need more of a rush in my work environment. So I took a job as a nurse in an emergency department—where you have to respond to new situations at a moment's notice.

I also had a passion for cardiac care. So eventually, I began working in cardiology as a nurse practitioner. I loved all of it.

But I had one nagging reservation. Over the course of my career in clinical medicine, it bothered me that most patients were getting sicker, not better. Western medicine's approach to acute and life-threatening disease and emergencies is undeniable, but it completely ignored the prevention of chronic disease.

By this time, I was married and had given birth to my first son. There was a problem, and I was worried. At around four months of age, despite being exclusively breastfed, he developed terrible eczema and was so miserable. He was prescribed various creams, none of which were helpful. I had to find something to cure it, and I wouldn't stop until I found it. Through dogged research, I discovered that his eczema was likely caused by a deeper, internal imbalance originating from poor gut health. I changed his diet to one of entirely unprocessed, natural and nutrient-dense foods. In fact, I made all the foods myself; nothing I fed him was commercially produced. Eventually, his skin cleared up. I also learned that he had life-threatening food allergies, which got me thinking that so many health problems originate with our food choices.

I continued to question the conventional medical approach to addressing and treating illness. Over time, I had become increasingly disillusioned with prescribing medication and more interested in the impact of nutrition on health and wellness. I wanted to know why my patients got chronically sick—so I investigated even more.

I became passionate about how I could help people prevent and treat illnesses before they even became chronic problems. I considered getting a doctoral degree but completed a wellness coaching certification instead. Then I found a functionally focused nutrition program that ignited my passion for helping my patients. I dove into the program and ultimately decided it was time to make a difficult choice—to leave my nurse practitioner's job and start my own private practice.

It was one of the best moves I've ever made. I eventually built a successful business and have now worked with thousands of women. I am asked to speak frequently on women's health and nutrition and intermittent fasting. I delivered two TEDx Talks, one in 2018 and a second in 2019. My second TEDx Talk, "Intermittent Fasting: Transformational Technique," went viral, received more than eight million views, and catapulted me to being a top thought leader in intermittent fasting and women's health. The response actually took me by surprise! I was humbled and profoundly grateful.

I'm also thankful for the extraordinary job I now have—guiding and caring for women like you who feel like they are at the end of their health rope. It is okay to feel like this, especially when you don't get the answers you want from the traditional medical establishment. You need and deserve a much different approach to health care—with safe, natural, and effective options that help you get the most out of your life. Providing these options and programs became my mission—my calling—in life.

I went on to create unique one-on-one programs and group programs that support and educate all of us on healthy aging—and how nutrition, lifestyle, mind-body practices, and other tools can chart a new course into what will be the healthiest, most fruitful stages of our lives.

There is such a hugely powerful relationship between the foods we eat and *when we eat them* and the improvements we see in our weight, health, and wellness. It is so empowering to know that if you listen to your body and give it what it needs, you can restore your health. My passion is and always will be to help women like you find wellness through the healing power of intermittent fasting and nutrition.

Your Journey

Which brings us to the journey you and I are about to take right now. IF:45 is your opportunity to engage in a transformative experience that will show you the power you have to lose weight and feel better—not in months from now, but in only forty-five days.

These forty-five days will be life-changing and lifestyle-changing for you. They will reset your metabolism and biology, rebalance your hormones, boost your energy, liberate you from cravings, drop pounds, and reverse chronic symptoms. They provide the solution to quickly and profoundly improving your health by changing just a few things: what you eat, when you eat, how you rest and recover, and a few more actions.

How you approach intermittent fasting will be unique for you. Every woman fits into a distinct biochemical profile, termed "bio-individuality." This is your own personal makeup of hormones, metabolism, and other specific health needs based on your age, gender, stage in life, and other factors. Because we are all unique, this program is designed around *your* bio-individuality—one of the main reasons IF:45 is different from other forms of intermittent fasting.

Over the past several years, I have guided more than a thousand women through this program. They have experienced profound success. They come to it for weight loss but stick with it for the antiaging and overall health benefits it offers. It becomes a lifestyle.

Here are some comments from women who participated in one of my recent Intermittent Fasting master classes:

"I have lost a total of eight pounds. Eighty percent of my love handles are gone. I feel more in tune with my body and can do extended fasts with no issues. I've been able to turn down pizza and candy at work. No longer do I feel fatigued—which has been huge for me. I have changed physically, emotionally, and mentally—in only three weeks."

"After I started the class, my sleep improved, my food choices were better, and I dropped seven pounds. For me—a fifty-eight-year-old menopausal woman, these benefits were life-changing. I finally realized that I was worth it, and the effort it takes to be healthy is worth it."

"I no longer feel hungry, but nicely satisfied. My only cravings are for wholesome food. My glucose readings have normalized. My sleep has improved, and I'm sleeping through the night. I have so much energy that I increased my walking intensity to a three-and-a-half-mile, fast-paced walk."

"I'm not addicted to sugar anymore. My thinking is clear. I'm not forgetting words mid-sentence, and I've dropped seven pounds."

"Intermittent fasting has given me time for a morning routine that involves walking, deep breathing, and enjoying green tea. I feel great and have been able to focus on building my online business with less anxiety. Since intermittent fasting, I have lost twenty pounds, reaching my goal weight, and my body is now more adapted to burning fat."

The IF:45 Plan

The program that these women followed so successfully—and so will you—is divided into three phases. Induction, a one-week preparatory phase, shows you how to clean up your pantry, eliminate gluten and dairy, stop snacking, and choose foods that kick-start fat-burning. With these simple actions, you will: See weight loss on the scales right away. Feel revitalized after removing foods that have been the source of your fatigue, bloating, and other gut issues, and foggy thinking. And begin to improve your health.

In the next phase, Optimization, you learn how to create your own fasting and feeding windows, select and time your macronutrients (protein, carbohydrates, and fats) based on whether you are cycling, going through perimenopause, heading into menopause, or coming out of it. If you loved what happened to your body the first week, you'll be overjoyed at your results in this phase: even more dramatic improvements in weight loss, cravings, sleep patterns, hormone balance, mental clarity, energy level, digestive function, and overall wellness.

After that, in the final phase, Modification, a one-week plan, I give you guidelines on advanced strategies, such as expanding your fasting window, varying your fasts, cycling carbohydrates, and more. All the benefits you've experienced so far continue in this phase—and are even more dramatic.

As I mentioned, you'll be hooked on this lifestyle and want to maintain it. And so I give you strategies for doing just that as you head into maintenance. IF:45 from this point forward becomes a natural and easy way of life!

This book can be a lifeline to help you feel better and live better. The benefits I've summarized so far can happen to you once you start following my program of intermittent fasting and stay true to its strategies.

In these pages, I go into detail about how intermittent fasting works and cover some fascinating material about how your body works hormonally. I take you through some basic science about how it affects your weight, various medical conditions, and your health in general.

You'll learn about what you should eat for best results—all backed by delicious recipes and easy-to-follow meal plans. We'll dive right into the specifics of the three phases, customizing the program for your stage of life and putting it into action. I'll be coaching you at every step along the way so that you're inspired, excited, and set up for success.

I suggest that you read this book sequentially to get familiar with the program, what you'll be doing—and why. Read everything with an open mind because I have some new information no one has told you before. Rest in the knowledge that you no longer have to resign yourself to the limiting belief that weight gain, fatigue, foggy thinking, and other health frustrations are normal functions of aging. They are not!

Give yourself grace as you follow the program, too, because there is tremendous flexibility built in. This is not a rigid plan, with a lot of dos and don'ts. It works with you, your unique chemistry, and your lifestyle. Once you get into the sync of intermittent fasting, you'll realize that it is a strategy you can harness for a lifetime.

I want you to know that I understand where you are. Remember, I was that woman desperate for answers at a time when traditional medicine was not enough. It's impossible to forget those days of feeling fat and demoralized, having no energy and fighting off the despair of defeat. But hear me—I'm uniquely positioned to support you and make sense of issues related to lack of energy, weight gain, food cravings, and more.

So—let me ask you: Are you ready for a transformation? If so, give yourself forty-five days, and you will lose weight, curb cravings, revitalize your body, and live to the fullest for the rest of your long and happy life.

How exciting is that?

Cynthia Thurlow

To view the 1 reference cited in this chapter,
please visit cynthiathurlow.com/references.

Part 1

Intermittent Fasting—

A Healthy Body and Healthy Hormones

Chapter 1

. . . .

Why Intermittent Fasting?

Something happens as you pass through your thirties and then your forties, with hints that your body is changing. You're gaining weight and fighting cravings. You're no longer bouncing out of bed the way you used to. You notice symptoms like bloating, poor sleep, brain fog, and mood swings. You're feeling old before your time, and just plain off. For the vast majority of us, these changes are agonizing, frustrating—and scary.

I get it. I really do, because of my own experience and my work with countless women like you. You're right to feel this way, and you're far from alone. But take heart. It is never too late to get healthier and regain your looks, health, mental clarity, and energy.

Heather is a good example. When she came to me at age fifty-four, having entered menopause four years prior, she was extremely frustrated. "Nothing ever worked for me," she said, in a low, dejected voice. "I've eaten mini-meals, I've counted calories, I've exercised like a maniac, but the weight just won't come off. I hate how this extra twenty pounds makes me feel so old and tired. Honestly, I've lost hope."

Heather had even resorted to taking a drug called phentermine. It is similar to an amphetamine, or "upper." It stimulates the central nervous system (nerves and brain), which accelerates your heart rate and blood pressure and curbs your appetite. It has a lot of scary side effects, ranging from mild to moderate: insomnia, headaches, dizziness, dangerously high blood pressure, chest pain, and shortness of breath.

This kind of struggle is simply not necessary. As Heather and I talked, I guided her through my philosophy about how best to lose weight and navigate menopause—and do it naturally, without the use of prescription drugs to lose weight. I explained to her that every part of my program is designed to ease her symptoms and get her back to feeling younger and more vibrant again.

Heather perked up and was ready to give the program her all. She adjusted her nutrition, and she slowly started intermittent fasting. Lo and behold, she lost ten pounds in the first eight weeks and kept going—without feeling deprived, hungry, or fatigued. Today, she has more energy and confidence than she ever thought possible at her age.

Like Heather, perhaps you have followed the usual pieces of advice: counting calories, eating small meals throughout the day, and having breakfast—all those lose-weight actions in which we've been schooled. Maybe you managed to drop a few pounds, but then you plateaued, yo-yo dieted, or couldn't keep the weight off.

Or maybe you acquired other worrisome symptoms. You just don't sleep as well, for example, and it takes longer to get going in the morning. Perhaps you have too many aches and pains. Or you can't think as clearly as you once could, or can't remember facts and events. It seems like your body is changing right before your eyes. These are terrible, exasperating predicaments, and it's easy just to give up, even though you want to feel fantastic again.

It never ceases to amaze me how much bad advice, under the guise of "wisdom," women are given about their health and weight loss, such as my personal fave: "Exercise more, eat less." That absolutely did not work for me and had the opposite intended effect. I gained weight, couldn't take it off, and generally felt unhealthy.

Important: Do not beat yourself up. You haven't failed; conventional wisdom has failed you. That "wisdom" centers around the following dogma:

Bad Dogma #1: Calories in, calories out—this is what matters.

If you're endlessly counting calories to drop pounds or manage your weight, you may be worrying about the wrong thing. It's the *quality* of the protein, carbohydrates, and fat we eat—not counting calories—that is an important key to fat loss, weight control, and health. This involves getting enough of the nutrients you need, including vitamins, minerals, and fiber, from your food choices.

Poor-quality foods—namely processed carbohydrates like candy, chips, soda, and commercially baked goods—contribute to weight gain and other symptoms, but not because they have a lot of calories. It's that they set into motion a series of reactions that make your body store fat. These foods break down rapidly into sugar. In response, your pancreas churns out higher levels of the hormone insulin. Insulin is like fertilizer for your fat cells. It tells your cells to grab calories and convert them into fat.

The other problem is that when we cut calories, the body fights back. Our metabolism slows down in order to keep food and energy around longer, and you begin to feel hungrier. This situation is a no-win for weight control, and it throws our hunger hormones leptin and ghrelin out of whack. (More about these hormones in upcoming chapters.)

Bad Dogma #2: Breakfast is the most important meal of the day.

Wrong! We have been repeatedly told that eating breakfast is a healthy thing to do, based on a series of bad research and breakfast cereal marketing. We've heard that skipping breakfast is a very bad habit and could lead to diabetes, weight gain, and other health problems.

Here's the deal: There's just not much evidence for any of this. In fact, an analytical review of thirteen clinical trials, published between 1990 and 2018, concluded that "the addition of breakfast might not be a good strategy for weight loss, regardless of established breakfast habit. Caution is needed when recommending breakfast for weight loss in adults, as it could have the opposite effect." The study also found that the breakfast skippers weighed less than the breakfast eaters.

Skipping breakfast is okay—and indeed, a good idea, with lots of benefits!

Bad Dogma #3: What we eat is more important than when we eat.

What you eat—healthy, wholesome, non-processed food—is absolutely vital. But it's also *when* you eat that really makes a difference. The "when" involves syncing your meals with your circadian rhythm—the complex physiological system that regulates your sleep-wake cycle and all the hormonal and metabolic processes involved in it. Intermittent fasting aligns with your circadian rhythm and metabolism to improve many health markers, including insulin sensitivity, cardiac risk factors, brain health, overall disease risks, and, last but not least, overweight and obesity.

A case in point about weight loss: Over a ten-week period, people who were instructed to both delay breakfast for ninety minutes and eat dinner ninety minutes earlier (thus changing the time frame in which they ate) lost twice as much body fat as those who were allowed to eat on their normal schedules, despite being allowed to eat whatever they wanted during feeding hours.

Timing is everything! It's the key to a healthy weight and protection from many diseases.

Bad Dogma #4: Eating small meals throughout the day promotes fat-burning and stabilizes blood-sugar levels.

How many times have you heard this one? Many people believe that eating multiple meals throughout the day bumps up metabolism, causing the body to burn more calories overall and keep hunger in check.

None of this is true. Some proof: Investigators at the University of Ottawa discovered that on a restricted-calorie diet, there was no weight-loss benefit to splitting calories among six meals rather than three.

Another study found that switching from three daily meals to six did not stimulate calorie-burning or fat loss. As for appetite control, there's no evidence that eating six meals a day curbs hunger; however, eating larger, less frequent meals will reduce your overall hunger and make you feel full.

A few years ago, I worked with a fitness competitor named Karen. Like many competitors in this sport, she had been brainwashed to believe that the only way to lose weight and be healthy was to eat six small meals daily. But this wasn't working for Karen. She was constantly preparing meals and became overly fixated on food—which often led to bingeing. I switched her over to my IF:45 plan, and she flourished. Karen told me: "Intermittent fasting changed my entire life and I've learned so much about food intake. My energy is through the roof, my skin is great, my sleep is awesome, and I'm not a prisoner to food anymore."

These antiquated dogmas have contributed to escalating rates of obesity, poor metabolic health, and disease that have reduced the quality of life for an entire generation and their offspring. Now at epidemic proportions, these health crises are affecting women in staggering numbers. According to data from the National Center for Health Statistics, the prevalence of obesity in women twenty years and older increased from 25.5 percent to 40.7 percent over the past few decades. A 2019 journal article suggested that by 2030, more than 25 percent of the general population in the United States will be defined as severely obese, which will be the most common obesity category for women. And obesity, of course, is linked to many life-crushing illnesses: heart disease, type 2 diabetes, many forms of cancer, and depression, to name just a few.

It is time to acknowledge that we need to do better in terms of solving the related issues of overweight, obesity, and ill health. Intermittent fasting is a huge part of the solution—and a clear path to health and weight freedom.

What Is Intermittent Fasting?

In simple terms, intermittent fasting is *eating less often*. You go without food for a period of time (your fast), and you eat within a "feeding window," a specific pocket of time designated for meals. In your feeding window, you enjoy protein, healthy fats, and non-starchy carbs, with no focus on calorie counting. You're deliberate about when you eat and when you fast, and you make a conscious decision to eliminate a meal or meals.

The three most widely used intermittent-fasting regimens are alternate-day fasting, in which you eat one day and fast the next; 5:2 intermittent fasting (fasting two days a week, eating the other five); and daily time-restricted feeding, in which you go twelve to sixteen hours or more, without food, including overnight, and then enjoy your meals within a designated window.

My IF:45 plan centers around time-restricted feeding, namely a 16:8 model (sixteen hours fasted, eight hours fed). It is the simplest to do, the most flexible—and the most appropriate plan for women of all ages. You can time your eating and fasting around your stage in life—cycling, perimenopause, and menopause and beyond—and organize it so that it keeps your hormones balanced. Plus, the fasting period isn't too long. You can start small and gradually stretch your window as your body gets used to fasting.

Unlike a lot of programs involving diets, time-restricted feeding has a higher adherence rate as shown in many studies. You can easily stick to it for as long as you want! My plan also lets you eat a wide variety of nutritious foods within that window. Above all, the 16:8 plan offers a long list of proven health benefits, especially for women.

The public perception is that intermittent fasting is something new—a novel way of dieting that has only come into vogue quite recently. What is often forgotten, though, is that intermittent fasting stretches much further back than living memory. In fact, it is very aligned with ancestral health patterns. Think about it: Our prehistoric and ancient relatives did not eat three square meals, spaced evenly apart, plus snacks. They did not have an endless, easy access to food like we do today. In fact, they probably didn't eat for long periods of time simply because food wasn't readily available. Based on the season or climate, they might have eaten several times during the day, whereas on other days, they may have had only one meal—or perhaps no food at all. I would thus argue that we're genetically primed for meal patterns with periods of fasting built in. It is our evolutionary heritage to fast intermittently!

Intermittent fasting is a powerful choice you can make for your health, your hormones, and your well-being as a woman. In fact, it is more powerful than any medicine I could prescribe. Eating in a shorter window and going without food for longer periods affords you some amazing benefits. Intermittent fasting:

Burns Fat

Many women in their thirties, forties, fifties, and beyond have spent years dieting, losing weight only to gain it back, again and again. Swings of ten, twenty, thirty, or more pounds from one year to the next are common, and a lot of us might have closets crammed with two wardrobes of large sizes and skinny sizes. This up-and-down routine is the definition of yo-yo dieting, which is dangerous to your health. An American Heart Association study reported that women who yo-yo diet have a higher number of risk factors for heart disease than women who have stabilized their weight over the years. Repetitive dieting is simply not a good practice! Yet it is a habit within your power to change—thanks to intermittent fasting.

A huge reason has to do with your hormones. Intermittent fasting activates certain key hormones in the body, many of which increase "lipolysis" (fat-burning), enhance your metabolic flexibility (the ability to use fuel appropriately—see below), help prevent your body from storing fat, and have many other positive effects on weight control and health. I'll cover these hormones in detail in upcoming chapters.

With your hormones in harmony, fasting helps accelerate your metabolic rate—which also allows you to maintain a healthy weight. And, according to one review, fasting can trim belly fat by 4 to 7 percent. As such, intermittent fasting is one of the most effective tools we have for losing weight.

Another factor has to do with the actual fat we carry. There are two types of fat tissue in your body: brown fat and white fat. Brown fat burns energy because it is plentiful in mitochondria, the powerhouses of our cells. White fat stores energy.

If you had to choose, which fat would you want more of? Brown fat, right? But it's not so simple. Brown fat is uncommon in adult humans. It's generally what makes up that cute "baby fat" in infants.

The good news is that scientists have recently discovered that we can turn our white fat into brown! Intermittent fasting can help make this happen.

This fortunate discovery was found in experiments with mice, who went on an every-other-day fasting plan. Another group of mice was allowed to eat anything they wanted, at any time. In the study, the researchers found that in the fasting mice, intermittent fasting changed the composition of their gut bacteria, and this stimulated the production of short-chain fatty acids (SCFAs) from the gut. This reaction turned white fat cells into brown fat cells and shifted fat storage to fat-burning, effectively reducing obesity and insulin resistance (a huge problem that causes diabetes).

Of course, this study was performed in our mice counterparts, and I take this into consideration when quoting studies. Mice, however, have metabolisms similar to humans, so the findings are pretty interesting nonetheless! The important message here is that intermittent fasting is a very effective way to burn fat—in positive ways.

Promotes Gut Health

Speaking of the gut: There are trillions of microorganisms living in your intestines, collectively called the microbiome. They break down food and synthesize nutrients, like B vitamins and vitamin K. They feed on dietary fiber and certain types of starch in foods, creating compounds that are vital to muscle function and disease prevention. Our gut bugs even influence our mood and thinking, sending signals between the brain and the digestive system. They do a lot of other things, too, like reducing inflammation and regulating your appetite—all of which impact your weight and health.

There are two main classes of weight-control bacteria in the gut: Bacteroidetes and Firmicutes. Body weight appears to be tied to a balance of the two. In many studies, some as recent as 2020, people with obesity had more Firmicutes and fewer Bacteroidetes than moderate-weight people. Yet there are other studies that have failed to establish this connection—so the jury is still out here.

Weight loss aside, feeding your gut bacteria the right stuff helps maintain the balance of good bugs to bad, protecting your health. But it's not only what you eat that impacts this balance, it's also when you eat. With fasting, there's a rapid expansion of good bacteria, for example.

Also, animal studies have shown that gut bacteria have their own circadian rhythm and are constantly cycling among different populations. Scientists who study the gut microbiome believe that when we're asleep and fasting overnight, one set of bacteria may thrive. When we're awake and eating, others flourish and take over. This cycle repeats itself every twenty-four hours.

Intermittent fasting also supports an important digestive mechanism called the migrating motor complex, or MMC. It controls stomach and small intestinal contractions in a cyclical pattern over a period of about two hours.

The MMC is also the "housekeeper" of the small intestine. It sweeps out any food particles from the small intestine and sends them to the large intestine. Working in cycles, the MMC only clears the small intestine during periods of fasting. It is actively shut down when we eat. So if you do a lot of snacking between meals, you may be compromising your MMC. Spacing out your meals through intermittent fasting improves MMC function.

Fasting also stimulates c-AMP, an energy molecule used by gut bacteria, especially those that make up your gut lining. This energy exchange further activates genes that protect your intestinal lining. All of this serves to improve its strength and integrity, so that bacteria, food particles, and toxins do not leak out (a syndrome called leaky gut) and cause health problems.

The good deeds of your gut bacteria don't end there. Intermittent fasting helps preserve the cells that produce serotonin. Serotonin is a vital, multi-purpose hormone in the body that affects mood and happiness. It is produced in a few places around your body, but mostly in the cells that line your gut—cells that are protected through intermittent fasting. Consequently, depression—something that affects more women than men, especially during midlife—has been shown to lessen through intermittent fasting.

Creates Metabolic Flexibility

You will frequently hear me use the term "metabolic flexibility" throughout this book. Simply put, it is the ability of your cells to switch between using carbohydrates and fat as a fuel source. If you are metabolically flexible, you can burn carbs when you eat them. You can burn fat when you eat it. Or you can burn fat when you're not eating at all (intermittent fasting). In short, your metabolism is flexible and can use whatever fuel is available, whether that fuel is from food or fuel already stored in your body.

During the Paleolithic Age, our ancestors were metabolically flexible by nature. Sometimes, there was plenty of food, while other days, it was scarce. Their bodies were necessarily proficient at burning fat during these periods of fasting.

Fast-forward to modern times, and things are vastly different. The abundance of processed foods has removed the necessity to burn body fat for fuel. What once was the norm has become the overwhelming minority.

Why is it important to be metabolically flexible?

Metabolic flexibility confers numerous health benefits: sustained energy, balanced hormones, fewer blood-sugar roller coasters, fewer cravings, and improved fat-burning, among others.

It also improves your exercise performance. Someone with good metabolic flexibility taps into fat for energy over carbs, and doesn't get fatigued as quickly.

In contrast, someone who's less metabolically efficient can't make the switch to burning fat as rapidly and will burn more glycogen (stored carbohydrates) and fatigue faster.

Intermittent fasting is one of the best ways to improve metabolic flexibility since you force your body to tap into fat stores—especially when you periodically decrease your carbohydrate intake.

Enhances Mitochondrial Health

The cells in your body contain several thousand organelles called mitochondria. They are cellular power plants that process oxygen and convert nutrients from food we eat into energy. Mitochondria produce 90 percent of the energy the body requires to function. If the mitochondria fail to generate enough energy, this can result in mitochondrial disease. Present at birth or brought on by an unhealthy lifestyle, mitochondrial diseases can inflict harm on almost any part of the body, including the brain, nerves, muscles, kidneys, heart, liver, eyes, ears, or pancreas.

Fasting keeps the mitochondria healthy and even creates new mitochondria—in a couple of different ways. Fasting increases "sirtuins," a family of proteins that ensure that your cells are working at their best. Sirtuins also regulate fat and glucose metabolism, fight chronic inflammation, boost energy levels, increase alertness, and repair damaged genetic material in cells. They are also involved in creating new mitochondria.

Sirtuins work in harmony with a molecule called NAD+, which is shorthand for nicotinamide adenine dinucleotide. It helps supply the energy sirtuins need to do their diverse jobs. NAD+ declines with age—one of the reasons we feel more tired, have brain fog, or have weakened immunity. Boosting NAD+ through strategies like fasting can fight aging and promote longevity.

Fasting also stimulates pathways that build new mitochondria, not just through sirtuins, but through the enzyme adenosine 5' monophosphate-activated protein kinase, or AMPK. It is known as the body's master regulator of energy metabolism and promotes fat-burning. Scientists believe that as we get older, AMPK activity significantly drops off. This is another reason why we experience changes in appetite, body weight, energy levels, and so forth. What really sparks AMPK activity is energy depletion—aka fasting.

Cleans Defective Cells

Fasting is the most effective way to trigger a process of cellular renewal called autophagy. Autophagy was discovered accidentally in the 1970s by a Belgian scientist, Christian de Duve, who was studying insulin at the time. It is a process by which your body cleanses cells by clearing out damaged, dysfunctional, or aging cells. It makes cells stronger, cleaner, and more efficient. You can think of it like your garbage disposal, breaking down refuse, eliminating it, and decluttering your kitchen. Autophagy, as coined by de Duve, gets its name from the Greek for "self" (auto) and "eating" (phagy).

In 1983, a researcher named Yoshinori Ohusmi, who was conducting experiments with yeast, discovered that genes regulate autophagy and, without those genes, the mechanism doesn't work and cells can't repair themselves. Both scientists were Nobel Prize winners.

It's fascinating to note that "cellular stress" boosts autophagy. An example of cellular stress is depriving cells of nutrients (fasting). Fasting thus kick-starts autophagy and improves the function of all your cells.

Autophagy is extremely important to antiaging and longevity. During autophagy, as your cells break down parts of themselves, they sequester these parts into vacuoles (small cavities within cells) and digest them. As a result, cells generate waste, mainly dead organelles, damaged proteins, and oxidized particles. Unless this waste is properly disposed of, it builds up and can become toxic to cells—an accumulation that promotes aging. Your skin looks older, your body slows down, energy dips, and your hormones become unbalanced and function poorly.

Fasting to the rescue! By accelerating the cleanup process, it helps turn back the aging clock. When you fast, autophagy ramps up after twenty-four to forty-eight hours on average and gets your body into ketosis. This is a normal state by which your body uses fatty acids for energy rather than glucose. Ketosis generates ketones, which become your primary source of fuel. At about twelve hours into fasting, you'll begin to move into the early stages of ketosis, in which your body stops relying on carbohydrates for fuel and begins burning your body fat stores instead.

In your feeding window, you can further activate autophagy by reducing the carbs you eat and including more healthy fats such as grass-fed butter, ghee, coconut oil, olives, extra-virgin olive oil, and avocados. Just be conscientious with portions. With too much dietary fat, your body will burn it rather than tapping into your fat stores for fuel.

Certain natural compounds in foods stimulate autophagy too: *apigenins* (parsley, celery, and many herbs); *fisetins* (strawberries, cucumbers, and onions); *indoles* (broccoli, Brussels sprouts, cabbage, and cauliflower); *quercetin* (capers, apple peels, and kale); and *resveratrol* (peanuts, grapes, red and white wine, blueberries, cranberries, and cocoa).

Besides these, other measures help promote autophagy: drinking coffee or herbal tea; eating medicinal mushrooms; supplementing with apple cider vinegar; spicing foods with curcumin, turmeric, and cayenne pepper; and taking berberine, a natural chemical found in several plants that is available as a dietary supplement.

From a lifestyle perspective, exposing yourself to heat and cold, working out using high-intensity interval training (HIIT), and getting high-quality sleep will also enhance autophagy.

Other Amazing Benefits of Autophagy

Besides its antiaging benefit, autophagy:

- Enhances metabolic efficiency by promoting mitochondrial health
- Prevents neurodegenerative disorders, such as dementia and Alzheimer's disease
- Reduces chronic inflammation, which underlies many diseases (see below)
- Strengthens the immune system by virtue of its ability to clean out bacteria and viruses
- Protects against cancer by suppressing chronic inflammation and repairing damaged DNA

Boosts Brain Health

As you incorporate intermittent fasting in your lifestyle, you're going to find yourself more mentally alert. Why is this? Many reasons! Fasting:

- Elevates levels of BDNF—brain-driven neurotrophic factor—a brain hormone that, when in short supply, causes foggy thinking, depression, and other mental health issues. Enough BDNF boosts serotonin, the brain chemical that helps you feel good.
- Assisting BDNF is beta-hydroxybutyrate (BHB), a ketone made by your liver naturally and the most abundant ketone in your body. BHB is produced at a faster rate during fasting or when you're following a low-carbohydrate diet. BHB helps your brain grow new brain cells and the connections (synapses) between them, provides energy to the brain for thinking, and protects the brain against neurodegenerative disorders, such as Alzheimer's.
- Increases the secretion of growth hormone, which in turn protects the brain, regenerates brain cells, and prevents brain cells from dying off.
- Protects against neurodegeneration by clearing out beta-amyloid plaques from the brain—protein tangles thought to be responsible for dementia—and prevents damage to brain tissue.
- Many people claim that the brain depends mostly on glucose for cognition and energy. In truth, though, the brain prefers to obtain its fuel from ketones like BHB, not from glucose. Too much glucose is toxic to the brain—a situation seen in the development of Alzheimer's. Ketones and BHB, in particular, make a much better fuel source. Plenty of research supports the fact that ketones benefit the brains of people with Alzheimer's, epilepsy, and traumatic brain injury.
- As noted, when you fast, your body produces ketones. Ketones provide about 50 to 75 percent of our brain fuel; the rest can be covered by the formation of glucose (gluconeogenesis). If you're experiencing brain fog, lack of productivity, or poor mental performance,

getting your body into ketosis might be a solution for you, and intermittent fasting helps make that happen. When your body starts producing ketones in a sufficient amount, your brain functions better and your mental clarity and performance will improve. Your brain loves to run on ketones!

Strengthens Immunity

During the COVID-19 pandemic, we heard a lot about immunity—the resistance of the body to infection by a disease-causing agent. Immunity is usually provided by our own immune system. This is our body's department of defense—an elaborate network of cells, tissues, and organs that band together to protect the body against invaders.

This remarkable defense works on different fronts. Some immune protectors create a barrier to stop germs from entering the body. Others attack germs that have slipped through that barrier. Failing that, still others mount an even stronger defense to destroy the invaders as they try to multiply.

For excellent health, we need a strong immune system, but there's no single way to do this. Instead, it takes a collection of healthy habits to fortify your immunity. One of these habits is intermittent fasting.

But wait a minute. Doesn't this seem counterintuitive? How can *not* taking in nutrients strengthen immunity?

Think about this: In nature, when animals get sick, they stop eating and instead focus on resting. I've seen this with my own pets, and you probably have too. This is a primal instinct to reduce stress on their internal system so that their bodies can rest and better fight off infection. All energy is then directed toward immunity and healing. We're the only species that accesses food during times of illness!

But when we periodically fast, some very important immune-building actions occur. Intermittent fasting:

- Helps the body flush out the digestive system and eliminate potentially harmful microorganisms from the gut—substances that could compromise immunity

- Allows the immune system to divert energy toward healing and fighting off invaders
- Reduces the release of inflammatory cytokines. Produced by the immune system, these are proteins that, when overproduced, can damage organs and tissues
- Kills off older and damaged immune cells and generates new ones
- Creates resistance to cellular toxins
- Improves the regeneration of intestinal stem cells, making them more functional and improving the integrity of the gut lining (Reduced adult stem cell function contributes to aging.)

The immune system is a true physiological wonder, with every part working together. Intermittent fasting is a terrific way to keep our immune forces healthy and strong.

Reduces Inflammation

Another powerful effect of intermittent fasting is that it reduces inflammation in the body. Inflammation comes in two types: acute and chronic. Acute inflammation is the body's initial response to injury, such as a cut, a wound, or an infection. After these are healed, the inflammation goes away.

Chronic inflammation is altogether different. It may be triggered by infections that don't go away, abnormal immune reactions that mistakenly attack healthy tissues, or conditions such as obesity. This kind of inflammation is serious. It has been linked to heart disease and stroke, cancer, and many other diseases.

But here's some promising news. Research shows that during fasting, inflammatory cells called monocytes are less active in the body, and fewer are released into the bloodstream. This means the inflammatory response is naturally dialed down.

Also involved in chronic inflammation are free radicals, highly destructive molecules that attack the cells of our bodies. They are generated by normal metabolic processes that go on within the body, poorly functioning mitochondria, or through exposure to toxins in food or our environment. They are both a cause and a result of inflammation. Cellular damage from free radicals instigates inflammation; and inflammation itself generates lots of free radicals. It's a vicious cycle, for sure.

Fasting helps prevent the release of free radicals and protects you from inflammation. This benefit has been observed in several studies, although it is not exactly clear how fasting squelches free radicals. Scientists believe that the switch between eating and fasting deprives cells of glucose (blood sugar), forcing them to tap into other sources of energy, like fatty acids. This cellular response is actually positive. It causes cells to remove poorly functioning mitochondria and replace them with *healthy* ones over time—a situation that cuts back the production of free radicals.

Slows Down Aging

This is one of my favorite aspects of intermittent fasting: It keeps us youthful! The reason has to do with the benefits I covered above—cellular renewal and regeneration through mitochondrial health and autophagy. But intermittent fasting fights aging in other ways, too, mainly by preventing life-shortening conditions like obesity, diabetes, cardiovascular disease, brain diseases, and even tumor growth. Bottom line: Intermittent fasting activates antiaging mechanisms and helps keep our bodies in a younger, healthier state.

Gives You Unexpected Gifts

After intermittent fasting became a huge part of my lifestyle, my life changed in unexpected ways. I had more time to reach my activity goals each day. I could go on more walks with my dogs Cooper, my Labradoodle, and Baxter, my Goldendoodle. It was easier to be consistent with my daily rituals like quality time with my family, relaxation, and sleep. I had additional time to organize my household and clean my house—activities I normally can't get to. Intermittent fasting simplified my life and opened doors of time to accomplish many important things. When you eliminate the number of meals you eat in a day or week, you'll experience these amazing benefits, too.

For many people, intermittent fasting also leads to spiritual awareness.

If you think about it, fasting is an ancient tradition practiced by most major religions for spiritual purposes, from self-discipline to enlightenment. The act of fasting draws you away from physical things like hunger, quiets your mind, promotes an inner stillness, and enhances a spiritual connection. Ultimately, fasting can be considered one more very important piece of your daily or weekly physical, mental, and spiritual routine.

Keep reading on, and we'll take a deeper dive into the subject of intermittent fasting and hormonal balance in the next chapter.

To view the 51 references cited in this chapter,
please visit cynthiathurlow.com/references.

Chapter 2
. . . .

Balance Your Master Hormones

As I studied intermittent fasting, using it in my own life and later with women in my practice, I was amazed by how it helped support hormonal balance. Hormones play such a pivotal role in our physical, emotional, even spiritual health and well-being that finding a natural option for nurturing them was a remarkable gift. With intermittent fasting, women reported greater strength and vitality and felt more empowered. Many were able to finally make positive changes in their lives in a variety of ways—changes in the way they responded to stress, navigated through the often challenging transitions of life, or renewed their passion for life. Intermittent fasting impacts our hormones in profound, exciting ways that go far beyond just weight loss.

Chris is a typical example of this. When this forty-five-year-old mom came to see me, she was desperate to improve her health. Chris had entered perimenopause—a stage of life sometimes called the "change before the change." She is one of millions of women between the ages of forty and fifty-five who experience irregular periods, sleep problems, fatigue, weight gain, and other symptoms that come with the beginning of the end of their reproductive years.

Chris was waking up every night and tossing and turning for hours— a common and troublesome problem among her age group. According to the CDC, among perimenopausal women, 56 percent are more likely than postmenopausal (40.5 percent) and premenopausal (32.5 percent) women to sleep fewer than seven hours, on average, in a twenty-four-hour period. She was so tired, she could barely function.

Chris was also having hot flashes, and her periods were heavy and irregular. Her annual physical and lab tests showed high blood pressure, high fasting glucose, and abnormal cholesterol readings. Her doctor wanted to put her on diabetes medication and statin drugs, because her health had deteriorated so quickly. Chris had no energy or desire to spend quality time with her children and felt "mama" guilt over it.

Everything going on with Chris had to do with imbalanced hormones—especially her three master hormones—insulin, cortisol, and oxytocin. They were out of balance, and her body and health were paying a significant price.

I reassured Chris that she was not stuck with her symptoms (and neither are you!). She enrolled in my IF:45 class. Within just two weeks, she was sleeping through the night. Her energy levels were through the roof. Even her digestion improved. After reducing her carbohydrate intake and adopting a strength-training program, Chris dropped ten pounds initially. Her blood sugar stabilized. Her periods became more regular and less heavy.

After six months of incorporating intermittent fasting into her lifestyle, Chris normalized her insulin levels and lost fifty pounds. Her blood pressure moved into a healthy range. Her lipid profile improved, too: lower triglycerides, higher HDL, and lower total cholesterol. Following this simple but immensely effective strategy, along with other supportive approaches, was life-changing for Chris, as it can be for you.

The Balancing Act

By definition, hormones are chemical messengers secreted into the bloodstream by various glands (referred to as the endocrine system). They then travel throughout the body, impacting any cell that contains a "receptor" for them. Receptors work like a lock-and-key mechanism. If the key fits the lock, then the door opens. If a hormone fits the cellular receptor, then the cell opens up and lets the hormone in.

All hormone production begins in the brain, with its different structures playing specific roles in concert with other organs and glands in your body. The actual command center for our hormones is the hypothalamus-pituitary-adrenal axis, or HPA, for short. The HPA regulates temperature, hunger, digestion, immunity, mood, libido, and energy. It also plays a huge role in governing our reactions to stress, either physical or mental.

The hypothalamus and the pituitary gland are situated in the brain. The hypothalamus specifically controls hunger, fatigue, sleep, and body temperature, and it secretes many different hormones. It partners with the pituitary gland, which communicates with the adrenals, thyroid, ovaries, testes, and other glands. The pituitary secretes hormones that impact metabolism, growth, sexual development, reproduction, blood pressure, and more.

When working properly, the HPA nurtures the delicate balance of our hormones in response to our biological needs, such as sleep, hunger, thirst, and other things we need for survival. On the downside, imbalances are created by poor sleep quality, stress, and the kinds of foods we consume, among other factors.

I'll be describing hormones individually over the next several chapters, but please know that they all should work together. Think of this like an orchestra: Each hormone is a unique instrument in which some are more dominant at times than others, but each must play the correct note. If one or more hormones produces more or less than required, this make the entire orchestra out of tune.

The Three Master Hormones

The hormonal orchestra has three conductors leading the performance: insulin, cortisol, and oxytocin. Any symptoms of hormonal imbalance you experience as you get older can often be traced back to these three.

Insulin, for example, impacts many other hormones, including the sex hormones estrogen, progesterone, and testosterone (we'll talk more about sex hormones in chapter 4). By balancing insulin, these hormones can return to more optimal levels, and your body can be healthier, stronger, and more resilient.

Cortisol must be balanced as well. Excessive levels affect estrogen, testosterone, and DHEA— dehydroepiandrosterone—a key vitality and antiaging hormone. A delicate balance exists between cortisol and thyroid hormones, too. If this balance changes, you may have health problems related to your thyroid. Excess cortisol can even interfere with insulin function.

Oxytocin, which we don't hear much about, is very much a multipurpose hormone. It helps keep cortisol in check and improves insulin problems. It can balance other hormones down the line, like progesterone, estrogen, and testosterone, as well as many others.

Each of these three hormones is crucial to the function of every other hormone in the body. When you get them in optimum balance, with the help of intermittent fasting, you can enjoy optimum health.

Insulin—Our Key Metabolic Hormone

One of our master hormones that responds exceptionally well to intermittent fasting is insulin. Secreted by the pancreas, insulin plays a very important role in your body and is key for blood-sugar (glucose) levels, metabolism, cell growth and repair, brain function, and weight control.

Importance

After you eat, your digestive system breaks down your food and partitions its nutrients so that they can be absorbed by the cells and tissues of your body. Carbohydrates in food are broken down into glucose, a type of sugar. That glucose is absorbed into your bloodstream and rises temporarily in response to food. Your pancreas then releases insulin to move the glucose into your cells. The more glucose you have in your blood, the more insulin your pancreas releases.

Under normal circumstances, insulin shuttles glucose into your cells for energy. It attaches to insulin receptors on cells throughout your body, instructing the cells to open up and let glucose in. It is thus vital that in-sulin work properly to move glucose into cells so that you remain meta-bolically flexible, meaning that your body can access whatever fuel is available—fat, glucose, or glycogen (stored glucose) for energy,

Once glucose enters your cells, your blood-sugar levels should go back to normal, usually within two to three hours. This cycle happens through-out the day. You eat a meal, glucose goes up, and insulin is secreted to bring it back down. Assisting insulin in this process is the hormone glu-cagon. It works with insulin to control blood-sugar levels and keep them within proper levels.

When you don't need glucose for energy, your body stores it in the liver and muscles in the form of glycogen. In simple terms, glycogen is made up of many connected glucose molecules stuck together. If you need a quick boost of energy or if your body isn't obtaining enough glucose from food, glycogen can be broken down into glucose for fuel. Also, insu-lin stimulates the creation and storage of glycogen from glucose.

The liver stores approximately 100 grams of glycogen. Muscle glycogen content varies from person to person, but it's approximately 500 grams, according to a 2011 study published in *Frontiers of Physiology*. How much is stored at any one time is closely related to your diet and how much storage glycogen you burn off through exercise.

Once glycogen stores max out, any excess glycogen is converted into a type of fat called triglycerides. This fat continuously circulates in the bloodstream to generate energy. Or it can get stored in your fat tissue.

Also, if you routinely eat more carbohydrates than your body can store, it has no choice but to deposit them inside the fat cells. Insulin di-rects this process, and it can cause weight gain over time. In this situation, insulin inhibits lipolysis (the breakdown of fat for energy). So yes—eating a big chunk of cheesecake could potentially end up on your butt, hips, or thighs.

Imbalances
With elevated insulin, mostly due to habitually eating too much sugar and highly refined carbs, you run the risk of developing insulin resistance.

This condition occurs when your cells become less receptive to insulin; their receptors won't open up to allow the hormone to move glucose from the bloodstream into the cell. Think of this as a delivery person (insulin) showing up at your doorstep with daily packages (glucose). Pretty soon, you're overwhelmed with packages, and you say, "Go away." That's a picture of insulin resistance.

It's a bad situation, too, because it can lead to type 2 diabetes, certain types of cancers, heart disease, and other illnesses, plus create conditions favorable for weight gain. Insulin resistance can worsen hot flashes and night sweats, which can be caused by low estrogen, fluctuating blood sugar, food sensitivities, and other factors.

Another factor involved in insulin resistance is chronic stress. Insulin and cortisol both increase if you're under severe stress. Cortisol prepares your body to cope with stress by *increasing blood sugar* to provide an energy source to muscles. To prevent glucose from being stored, cortisol slows down insulin production. This allows glucose to be used immediately during stressful times. But when cortisol levels stay chronically elevated, *the body can remain in an insulin-resistant state.*

People with insulin imbalances are not metabolically flexible. As I noted earlier, this means the body can't efficiently switch between burning carbs and burning fat to produce fuel for energy. Research indicates that those who suffer from insulin resistance, prediabetes, or type 2 diabetes are typically metabolically inflexible. Fortunately, this problem can be resolved with intermittent fasting, proper nutrition, and other lifestyle changes.

Insulin imbalances also make women susceptible to:

- Estrogen dominance, in which your body has an imbalance in excess estrogen. This can show up as things like premenstrual syndrome (PMS), endometriosis, ovarian cysts, heavy menstrual bleeding, benign breast disease, and accelerated aging. (For more on estrogen dominance, see pages 50–51.)
- Appetite changes that result in almost uncontrollable cravings for sweets and carbohydrates. Cravings are generally the result of blood-sugar instability due to insulin resistance. Every time blood

sugar drops rapidly, certain cells in the brain send powerful signals to the hypothalamus, which then stimulate food cravings and near-constant urges to eat.

- Insulin resistance also upsets the balance of two "happy hormones"—dopamine and serotonin. Both are responsible for normal hunger cues, but when they're imbalanced, you're likely to feel hungry more often.

- Polycystic ovary syndrome (PCOS), a hormonal disorder in some women of reproductive age. According to the Mayo Clinic, the exact cause of PCOS is unclear, but it may be triggered by excess insulin, heredity, inflammation, and overproduction of male hormones. Common symptoms include infrequent or prolonged menstrual periods, inability to conceive, and cysts in the ovaries. Your health care provider can diagnose PCOS using a system called the Rotterdam criteria, based on a spectrum of symptoms, ranging from mild to severe, with many variations in between.

- Fluid retention. Ever wonder why you feel bloated and look bloated? One reason can be attributable to higher insulin levels. These cause your kidneys to hold on to salt and water, and your body retains fluid. One solution is to lower insulin levels by restricting carbohydrates. When you cut back on carbs, your body loses salt (sodium) in your urine—a process called "diuresis." With diuresis, there's less bloating.

- Diuresis is partially the reason for the quick weight loss that occurs within the first several days after starting a low-carb diet. This has to do with glycogen and its association with water retention. Each gram of glycogen holds 3 to 4 grams of water. So, as your body burns into the glycogen stores, the water attached to the glycogen is lost, resulting in the phenomenon commonly known as "losing water weight."

Intermittent Fasting and Insulin

Following an intermittent fasting lifestyle promotes healthier insulin levels. Here's why: Food is the impetus for insulin secretion. If you are constantly eating, you are constantly secreting insulin. When insulin levels remain high, you store more fat and potentially develop insulin resistance and metabolic inflexibility. But when you fast, your body lowers its insulin levels. Your cells can then become more insulin sensitive, and your body can use up stored sugar and then, ultimately, use fat as fuel.

In a 2018 study, researchers found that fasting *reversed* insulin resistance and permitted patients to wean off insulin therapy without altering their blood-sugar levels. The relationship between insulin and fasting also helped patients shed pounds and reduced their waist circumference.

Another study that analyzed intermittent fasting and insulin resistance found that participants who fasted saw a 3 to 6 percent reduction in their blood sugar, and a 20 to 31 percent decline in their insulin levels. Researchers involved with the study suggested that fasting is equally as effective as traditional calorie reduction to accelerate weight loss, protect heart health, and prevent type 2 diabetes.

With intermittent fasting, your body has extended periods of time with lower insulin levels. Lots of benefits kick in, including fat-burning.

Cortisol—the Major Stress Hormone

When you're stressed out, your body is under attack. It prepares to either *fight* the perceived stressor, *flee* from it, or *freeze*—a response governed by your sympathetic nervous system, or SNS.

The SNS is activated by the hypothalamus, which sends signals to the adrenal glands to pump the hormone epinephrine (also known as adrenaline) into the bloodstream, directing blood to your muscles, heart, and other vital organs. Your pulse rate and blood pressure accelerate, and you begin to breathe more rapidly.

If the threat continues, the hypothalamus dispatches corticotropin-releasing hormone (CRH). It makes its way to the pituitary gland and triggers the release of adrenocorticotropic hormone (ACTH). This hormone heads to the adrenal glands, where it prompts them to churn out cortisol. Cortisol frees up blood sugar to provide strength and energy to defend yourself. It also elevates your blood pressure in order to increase the supply of oxygen and nutrients to all parts of your body.

When the threat passes, cortisol levels usually fall, and your body should return to its normal state, thanks to an opposing system—the parasympathetic nervous system (PNS). It takes over and calms your body down after the danger has passed.

Think of both systems like this: The SNS is like the gas pedal in your car—it accelerates the stress response—while the PNS acts like the brake pedal to stop the stress response.

But from what I often see, most people are living their lives in a state of perpetual fight-or-flight mode due to chronic stress, and this means that their sympathetic nervous system is in overdrive. Jumping into the act is a part of the brain called the amygdala. It is often referred to as the "lizard brain" because it is about all a lizard has for its primitive brain function. The amygdala overrides the prefrontal cortex "thinking and reasoning" part of the brain—which means we can no longer make sound rational decisions. All the more reason to get stress under control!

Importance

Cortisol is important to our overall health and well-being, and we can't live without it. Besides preparing us for stress, cortisol has other vital functions. Cortisol:

- Acts as a natural anti-inflammatory if your body is assaulted by an injury, arthritis, or allergy
- Stimulates the immune system
- Boosts alertness, concentration, mood, and other cognitive functions
- Regulates appetite and fights cravings
- Guards cardiovascular health
- Aids in fertility
- Helps muscles respond to exercise

Imbalances

Cortisol is clearly a beneficial hormone. However, it has a dark side when chronically elevated by unresolved stress (perceived or otherwise)—like working for a bad boss or struggling financially or staying in an unhealthy relationship. These persistent stressors flood your system with cortisol, which then becomes toxic to your body. Chronically elevated cortisol also interferes with the production of other hormones, including insulin, oxytocin, and our sex hormones—progesterone, estrogen, and testosterone. If we remain in a fight-or-flight state with an overactive SNS, our bodies can wear down. All kinds of metabolic turmoil kick in, including high insulin, chronic inflammation, lowered immunity, stress-related digestive problems, and many other health problems.

One of the biggest concerns with excessive cortisol has to do with weight gain and obesity. Cortisol drives weight gain in three ways.

First, chronic elevation of cortisol can result in "visceral fat" storage. This is a fat that hides out under the white fat in your midsection and pads vital internal organs. Its purpose is to protect organs like your liver and intestines. You can't always see or feel it, but too much of it can increase inflammation, leading to serious health problems such as insulin resistance, diabetes, heart disease, and breast cancer.

Cortisol expedites the accumulation of this fat by mobilizing triglycerides from storage and relocating them to visceral fat cells. Within these fat cells are enzymes that create even more cortisol, adding insult to injury since the adrenal glands are already secreting more cortisol.

Triglycerides are drawn like a magnet to visceral fat because we have forty times more cortisol receptors there than in the fat just under our skin—subcutaneous fat—fat that you can pinch between two fingers. The quantity of cortisol receptors also explains the phenomenon of "cortisol belly"—fat around the waistline that develops as a result of too much stress.

Second, high blood-sugar levels create higher cortisol levels that in turn promote the storage of visceral fat. Excess cortisol also stimulates "gluconeogenesis." This is a process by which your body breaks down protein reserves into glucose to be used as fuel or for storage. It also mobilizes the fat from its storage elsewhere in the body and moves it to visceral fat. When you're constantly stressed out, it's easy to see how your body gains visceral fat.

Third, cortisol boosts your appetite and cravings for high-carbohydrate, sugary foods, as shown in various studies. A study at the University of California, San Francisco, demonstrated that premenopausal women who secreted more cortisol during and after simulated stress-provoking situations in the lab chose to eat more foods high in sugar and fat. Giving into cravings leads to weight gain.

Although elevated cortisol causes the most problems, cortisol levels can be too low. Cortisol deficiency occurs when the adrenal glands do not produce enough cortisol, usually due to Addison's disease or a diseased pituitary gland.

Intermittent Fasting and Cortisol

When discussing fasting and cortisol, it's important to explain that fasting is a "hormetic stressor"—a beneficial type of stress that creates a reaction in the cells to better prepare your body for stronger stressors in the future.

Even so, if you're under a lot of stress, fasting is not a good idea—at least not now—because fasting does not lower cortisol but potentially raises it.

I thus urge women who want to do intermittent fasting to get factors such as sleep, nutrition, and stress management under control prior to starting my IF:45 plan. When you do that, you gain all the benefits of intermittent fasting, including cortisol balance. Throughout this book, you'll learn how to set your lifestyle to successfully support intermittent fasting with a variety of self-care strategies.

Oxytocin—the Mother Hormone

Maybe you've heard of oxytocin? It is our hormone of connection, love, and bonding. Oxytocin is produced by the hypothalamus and stored and secreted into the bloodstream from the pituitary gland. It is also released from other tissues, including the brain, uterus, placenta, ovaries, and testes. There are even oxytocin receptors on cells in your digestive tract. This hormone stimulates gastric juices and hormones so your body can absorb more nutrition. It is a rather amazing hormone with the potential to improve our physical, mental, and emotional health when maintained at its correct level.

Importance

Oxytocin is released during breastfeeding and helps a mother bond to her newborn. Levels also soar with sexual intimacy, particularly during orgasms.

Oxytocin fluctuates throughout your menstrual cycle, peaking around the time of ovulation, when an egg is released in anticipation of fertilization. Not surprisingly, you might feel a little more amorous and frisky as a result, which may be an attempt to help increase chances of conception and pregnancy. Along with estrogen and progesterone, oxytocin then decreases during the luteal phase of your cycle, right after ovulation, and might be why you have mood swings at this time.

As for its relationship with insulin, oxytocin makes our cells more insulin sensitive. That is a good thing, because it helps create more metabolic flexibility so that cells use fuel more efficiently.

Oxytocin counteracts and lowers cortisol, too, helping you manage stress. If low in oxytocin, we can feel more stressed, less connected to others, or not as confident about ourselves. But at stable levels, oxytocin makes us happy and peaceful, charges up our sex life and passion, promotes health and healing, and helps us stay and feel more youthful.

In recent years, exciting new discoveries have been made regarding oxytocin's effect on other aspects of health. One has to do with diabetes and weight. One group of researchers discovered that oxytocin reversed insulin resistance and improved glucose tolerance in obese mice. With improved insulin function, weight loss followed. They also studied a group of obese people without diabetes. They found that good cholesterol (HDL) went up and bad cholesterol (LDL), weight, and after-meal blood glucose levels all went down with oxytocin.

Oxytocin might also prove to be a strong ally in the control and prevention of osteoporosis. At the ages twenty-five to thirty, women start gradually losing bone mass. As a result of changes in the amount of estrogen in the body, this bone loss accelerates after menopause. Scientists at São Paulo State University in Brazil showed that when oxytocin was administered to female rats at the end of their fertile period, the hormone reversed certain triggers of osteoporosis. Those triggers included diminishing bone density, loss of bone strength, and a deficiency of substances required for bone formation.

Imbalances

Imagine a world where you couldn't bond to your newborn or feel connected to loved ones or had no interest in a monogamous relationship. That's a world without oxytocin. Pretty devastating, right?

The importance of oxytocin cannot be overstated. With oxytocin, there's no in between—oxytocin is either secreted at a level where it performs its amazing work, or its absence will be felt with distressing symptoms.

Signs of low oxytocin include:

- Little or no pleasure in sex
- Inability to attach in relationships
- No interest in social interaction
- A feeling of being stressed out on an ongoing basis
- Depression and anxiety

These are just a few symptoms, and they're not good for your overall mental and physical health.

Fortunately, oxytocin has so many good things going for it that we obviously want to get more of it, right? There are many ways to boost oxytocin besides mother-child bonding and sexual intimacy: cuddling, hugging, doing yoga, meditating, getting a massage, or playing with your children or your pets. Even going shopping can release it!

Intermittent Fasting and Oxytocin

Enhancing your oxytocin levels can help you fast more easily and longer—by suppressing hunger and cravings. Studies have shown that oxytocin helps dieters stay fuller longer and experience fewer between-meal cravings.

In one study, researchers showed images of high-calorie foods to ten overweight and obese men. Parts of the brain involved in eating for pleasure lit up as they viewed the images. The subjects were then given either a dose of oxytocin or a placebo. In the men given oxytocin, brain activity in those areas weakened, meaning that the hormone reduced their cravings for high-calorie foods.

Of course, we definitely need more science on the link between food cravings and oxytocin, especially in women. But here's what I suggest in the meantime: When you fast, *get connected* with hugs, kisses, and other forms of bonding at intervals during the day. I say that because the presence of our bonding hormone starts dissipating in three- to five-minute intervals, so you'll need little doses in your day to keep oxytocin at healthy levels.

Clearly, the master hormones have a significant influence on your health, and they are continually in flux depending on your stage in life—as are *all* hormones. From a physical and emotional standpoint, all of your hormones are what make you who you are. And they definitely make us women, and men, men! I'm not exaggerating when I say that hormones are vital to every single function in your body. You cannot live without them being properly balanced. My IF:45 plan will help you restore that balance.

To view the 16 references cited in this chapter,
please visit cynthiathurlow.com/references.

Chapter 3

. . . .

Trigger Your Weight-Control Hormones

"No matter what I do, I can't lose weight."

This is one of the most common concerns I hear from my patients and clients. They are intensely frustrated with the unwelcome changes in their body as they age, especially feeling out of sorts and frumpy. They don't like the way they look. They're tired of being told, "You're getting older. There's nothing you can do so just live with it."

But despite all this, they are very motivated to start intermittent fasting in order to shed weight. I totally understand. After all, that's why I gave it a try—to get rid of unflattering weight that crept onto my body during perimenopause.

The fact is, as we get older and our hormones shift, our shape changes, favoring more fat over muscle. It has been estimated that the average American woman puts on fifteen pounds between ages thirty and seventy—without even trying or changing her diet. We lose muscle (unless we strength train). Fat builds up and shifts to places like our waist, hips, and thighs. Our bodies sag where we used to be perky and toned.

We so desperately want to look and feel our best!

If we can get there—and we can—there are other amazing benefits to enjoy. I like to remind women that the battle to keep weight down goes beyond appearance and fashion. With excess body fat, you run the risk of becoming insulin resistant or even diabetic, getting high blood pressure, developing cardiovascular disease, or suffering from osteoarthritis—all associated with obesity. Staying lean and fit means staying healthy.

What is the best way to accomplish that? You and I both know that there is plenty of advice out there on how to do this, what to eat, how to exercise—some plans are medically sound, others are quick fixes and potentially dangerous fads. Yes, you have to watch what you eat, and you must stay active. Both will get you started. But they are not enough.

What it takes is to correct the hormonal issues underlying the weight gain and fat redistribution. Any and all hormonal imbalances make it tough to lose weight and keep it off, and will only increase your risk of obesity.

Diet and exercise don't solve the problem alone. You must balance your hormones. Any program that does not address your hormones—particularly your weight-control hormones—does you a disservice and you won't get permanent results. When certain hormones become unbalanced or decline with age, they encourage weight gain and trigger secondary problems related to hormonal deficiencies.

Now for the good news: Pairing intermittent fasting with better nutritional and lifestyle choices does more than typical diets will ever do. This combination heals and rebalances hormones, corrects deficiencies and metabolic problems, and gets you to an ideal, stable weight and with it, all the life-enhancing benefits I talked about in chapter 1.

The Weight-Control Hormones

In truth, all hormones impact your weight, considering that they affect metabolic rate, appetite, muscle tissue, the ability to use glucose for energy, stress levels, sleep, and water retention. You already know about some weight-affecting hormone issues, like cortisol and insulin imbalances. But other, more subtle ones are keeping you from the body you want. Managing these will help your weight, shape, and appetite.

Leptin and Ghrelin—the Hunger Hormones

Many people I've worked with think they'll get unbearably hungry during a fast or that they'll feel weak or shaky, or will not be mentally clear. Trust me: You should not. This is because intermittent fasting helps to control two of your main hunger hormones: satiety-boosting leptin and appetite-boosting ghrelin.

Importance—Leptin

Known as the "satiety hormone," leptin was discovered in 1994, and scientists believed that it could hold the keys to unlocking the physiology of obesity and weight gain because it plays a role in reducing hunger. This hormone is produced mostly in your white fat cells (adipocytes), as well as in brown fat tissue, ovaries, skeletal muscle, the lower part of your stomach, and a few other places.

After you eat a meal—and feel like pushing yourself away from the table—that's leptin at work. If leptin is working properly, you can eat to the point of satisfaction and not crave any more food. Also, by regulating energy and food intake, leptin helps you maintain your weight.

Since leptin was discovered, our understanding of its role in the body has expanded. Instead of just a "hunger hormone" that suppresses appetite, leptin:

- Burns blood fats (triglycerides) for fuel
- Helps turn white fat into brown fat
- Governs fat storage
- Affects exercise (moderate activity can improve leptin sensitivity)
- Is involved in bone formation
- Regulates immune and inflammatory responses
- Helps create new blood cells and new blood vessels
- Assists in wound healing
- Initiates puberty
- Controls blood pressure, heart rate, thyroid function, and our menstrual cycle

Imbalances—Leptin

In some people, the brain struggles to detect leptin. The "I'm full" response doesn't register. This is called leptin resistance and is a type of hormonal imbalance. It is often accompanies metabolic inflexibility and can create or contributes to insulin resistance. And it leaves you ravenous for more food and increases your cravings for sugary carbohydrates.

There's also a cycle involved: The more you eat, the more you put on additional fat, and the less sensitive your body becomes to leptin. Leptin resistance may be one major reason why you gain weight and have such a hard time losing it.

There are other side effects. Leptin resistance compromises your thyroid health, possibly slowing your metabolism. It elevates your blood pressure, which is not good for your cardiovascular health. It worsens mood disorders like anxiety and depression, and sets in motion many other problems.

What causes leptin resistance? Some of the usual suspects are:

- Obesity
- Chronically elevated insulin levels
- Inflammation in the hypothalamus
- A diet high in inflammatory foods, especially sugar
- Poor sleep and insomnia
- Lack of exercise

Importance—Ghrelin

Ghrelin is known as the "hunger hormone." Long after your last meal exits your stomach, and between meals, ghrelin steps in like your mom or grandmother who's always telling you to "eat something."

Ghrelin stimulates your appetite, increases food intake, and promotes fat storage. According to the Society for Endocrinology, adults who were given ghrelin increased their food intake by 30 percent!

Ghrelin is produced and released mainly by your stomach, with small amounts also secreted by your small intestine, pancreas, and brain. It is regulated by the parasympathetic nervous system (PNS), which is highly involved in digestion. After ghrelin stimulates your hunger, and you satisfy that hunger with a meal, the PNS instructs the digestive system to "rest and digest," and concentrations of ghrelin subside.

Ghrelin also activates the release of growth hormone, which breaks down fat tissue and promotes the growth of muscle tissue. In addition, ghrelin protects the cardiovascular system and helps control insulin release.

Imbalances—Ghrelin

Ghrelin levels rise significantly when you go on a weight-loss diet. The longer you diet, the more your levels will increase—which is one reason why typical diets don't work in the long run. Case in point: One study of dieters found a 24 percent increase in ghrelin levels on a six-month diet. So if you want to shed pounds, lowering your ghrelin levels can be beneficial.

Ghrelin levels are also high in people who have the eating disorder anorexia nervosa. This may be a defense mechanism by the body to stimulate food intake and thus encourage weight gain.

Because ghrelin is produced primarily by the stomach, weight loss after gastric bypass surgery may trigger impaired ghrelin secretion.

This entire hormonal hunger system serves a purpose, and most of the time it works well. But any alteration in the ghrelin-leptin balance leads to increased appetite, cravings for sweets and simple carbs, overeating, emotionally driven eating, and a slower metabolism.

Intermittent Fasting and the Hunger Hormones

Most of the time you spend intermittent fasting is overnight while you're asleep. Fortunately, your leptin levels rise during sleep. This means that your brain is communicating to your body that much less energy is required during sleep than when you're awake.

As for fasting and leptin levels, researchers have studied what happens to people during Ramadan. This is the month when Muslims fast by abstaining from food or drink during daylight hours. In one study, women fasting during Ramadan showed a big increase in leptin, signifying that they felt satisfied during the fast.

When your stomach is empty from fasting, you'd think that more ghrelin would be secreted, making you hungry. Surprisingly, this isn't true. Fasting actually turns off ghrelin and makes you *less* hungry.

In one study, people went on a thirty-three-hour fast, in which ghrelin was measured every twenty minutes. One of the big findings was that ghrelin levels stayed stable throughout the fast. In other words, not eating for thirty-three hours made you no more or less hungry than when you began. Whether you ate or did not eat, your hunger level stayed the same.

In another study, over three days of fasting, ghrelin gradually decreased. The participants were far less hungry, despite not having eaten for three days.

But you don't have to go that long. A study in the journal *Obesity* looked at the 16:8 fasting method and found that after four days of eating within an eight-hour window, fasters had lower ghrelin levels overall and said their hunger level was pretty low.

One reason for this is that when you're not eating, you're not secreting insulin, and your blood sugar isn't going up and down all day—so you don't feel hunger or cravings.

The upshot of research involving hunger hormones is that hunger does not increase to unmanageable levels when you fast. Rather, it decreases—which is exactly what you want. You want to eat less and feel more full.

Intermittent fasting, unlike caloric restriction, is the way to do that. Let me emphasize, too, that in addition to intermittent fasting, it's vital to get a good night's sleep—consistently. The reason is that poor-quality sleep increases ghrelin. So if you're not sleeping well, you'll walk around hungry all day, craving processed carbohydrates such as cake, cookies, candy, and other forms of junk food.

Meet Some Other Hunger Hormones

Other hormones play a supporting role in hunger and appetite:

- Neuropeptide Y (NPY). Found mostly in the hypothalamus, NPY delays the feeling of fullness throughout a meal. Leptin helps to stop the firing of NPY, shutting off the signal to eat.
- Peptide YY (PYY). This hormone is manufactured in your intestines after you eat. It then enters your bloodstream and travels to the hypothalamus, where it hinders NPY, decreasing your appetite.
- Cholecystokinin (CCK). The first satiety hormone to be discovered, CCK is secreted in the gastrointestinal tract, especially in the small intestine. CCK rises quickly after you eat, and it triggers the initial release of PYY.
- Glucagon-like peptide-1. Abbreviated GLP-1, this hormone is secreted by your digestive tract after you eat. It acts as a satiety hormone, helping you feel full.
- Adiponectin. This hormone helps improve insulin sensitivity and balance blood-sugar levels so that you do not feel hungry and overeat. It is also involved in fat-burning.

Glucagon—the Fat Releaser

Secreted by the pancreas, glucagon works with insulin to regulate blood sugar (glucose) and keep it stabilized. Its job is to prevent levels from falling too low, and it does this mainly by converting stored carbohydrates in the liver into glucose. If your brain gets the message that your body needs food, it secretes glucagon. Glucagon is also involved in burning fat. Whereas insulin creates fat, glucagon breaks down fat and releases it so your body can use it for energy on a long-term basis.

Importance

To prevent low blood glucose levels, glucagon acts on the liver in three ways:

First, it converts stored carbohydrates (glycogen) in the liver into glucose, so that this fuel can enter the bloodstream for energy. This process is termed glycogenolysis.

Second, it stimulates the production of glucose from amino acids—a process called gluconeogenesis, mentioned earlier.

Third, it cuts back on glucose usage by the liver. This in turn means more glucose is available to the bloodstream in order to maintain proper blood-sugar levels.

As noted, glucagon is a fat-burning hormone, too. It stimulates the breakdown of fat for energy when glucose is low.

Imbalances

Unlike most hormones, imbalances of glucagon are rare. But if you have wide and frequent swings in your blood glucose levels, your body may not be regulating glucagon properly. Signs of abnormal glucagon levels include hypoglycemia, or low blood sugar, and the dizziness, faintness, fatigue, and confusion that often accompany it.

Intermittent Fasting and Glucagon

Intermittent fasting keeps insulin levels low when you are metabolically flexible. Glucagon steps in to stabilize your blood-sugar levels and keep them from dipping too low. It also puts your body in a fat-burning mode.

If, as part of your feeding window, you restrict carbohydrates and increase protein, you further stimulate the release of glucagon. The net effect of intermittent fasting and a low-carb, high-protein feeding window is to increase glucagon so that it can burn fat, keep blood sugar steady, and prevent your body from overproducing insulin (which means less fat storage).

Growth Hormone—the Youth Hormone

Growth hormone (GH) is produced and secreted from the pituitary gland. GH impacts nearly every cell in your body and stimulates the release of growth factors in the body. It also helps other hormones enter cells and work more efficiently. GH is thus important for growth, cell regeneration, and cell repair. It is often considered to be the fountain of youth because it has been shown to slow the aging process.

Importance

GH helps to maintain, build, and repair healthy tissue in the body, particularly muscle mass. This is important because muscle promotes metabolic flexibility, burns fat, and maintains a leaner body composition (a more desirable proportion of muscle to body fat). GH also:

- Improves the elasticity of your skin
- Builds greater bone density
- Enhances your immune system
- Gives you more energy and stamina
- Increases mental clarity
- Boosts your mood

GH is typically secreted before waking up in the morning along with cortisol and adrenaline. This collective response signals your body to increase the availability of glucose for fuel so that you have energy to start your day.

Imbalances

Like so many hormones, GH peaks in your early twenties and then starts a downward slide as you get older. By the time you hit fifty, you have about half the amount you had earlier in life. And it continues to decline from there. The major side effects are increased body fat, lower lean muscle, and loss of bone tissue.

This natural slowdown has sparked interest in prescribing synthetic growth hormone as a way to delay some of the changes linked to aging, such as decreased muscle and bone mass.

Normally, synthetic growth hormone is prescribed to children who have certain conditions that cause failure to grow normally. But according to the Mayo Clinic, if this drug is taken by children or adults with normal growth, who do not need man-made growth hormone, serious unwanted effects may result. These include the development of diabetes; abnormal growth of bones and internal organs such as the heart, kidneys, and liver; atherosclerosis (narrowing and hardening of the arteries due to buildup of plaque [fats] in the artery wall); and high blood pressure. Fortunately, however, there are natural ways to increase GH in your body.

Boost GH Naturally

Along with fasting, you can support GH production in other ways:

- Lose belly fat (intermittent fasting can help). Those with higher levels of belly fat likely have impaired GH production and an increased risk of disease.
- Eliminate refined sugar. It increases insulin, and higher insulin levels are associated with lower GH levels.
- Avoid food prior to bedtime. Late-night eating can spike insulin, interfering with nighttime production of GH.
- Optimize your sleep, since GH is released overnight.
- Exercise at a high intensity with HIIT or Tabata training.

Intermittent Fasting and GH

One of the most promising ways to naturally elevate GH is through intermittent fasting. When you fast, your body produces more GH (and less insulin). In one study, in which people fasted for two days, the blood levels of growth hormone increased as much as fivefold! Higher levels of this hormone activate fat-burning, boost muscle gain, make you feel young again, and have numerous other benefits.

Norepinephrine—a Stress Hormone That Burns Fat

Also known as noradrenaline, norepinephrine is both a hormone, produced by the brain and adrenal glands, and a neurotransmitter, a chemical messenger that sends signals across nerve endings.

Together with other hormones such as cortisol, norepinephrine helps the body respond to stress. It is involved in our primitive fight-or-flight response that prepares our body for either fighting or escaping and was a lifesaving response for our ancient ancestors when they had to flee from saber-toothed tigers and other predators. While it may not be a vicious saber-toothed tiger chasing us, there are many figurative "saber-toothed tigers" looming in our minds—financial problems, work-related stress, relationships gone bad, and others. Norepinephrine and other stress hormones help us respond to these "threats."

Importance

In the brain, norepinephrine helps regulate attention, alertness, vigilance, and anxiety. It also tells your body to release fatty acids from fat cells and increase blood sugar to supply more energy to the body.

Together with adrenaline, norepinephrine accelerates your heart rate, causing your heart to pump more blood. Norepinephrine also plays a role in the sleep-wake cycle, helping you to wake up and get focused for the day.

Imbalances

Poorly balanced norepinephrine levels are associated with depression, anxiety, post-traumatic stress disorder, and substance abuse. Low levels can cause fatigue, lack of concentration, attention deficit hyperactivity disorder (ADHD), and possibly depression.

Intermittent Fasting and Norepinephrine

When you fast, your nervous system dispatches norepinephrine into your bloodstream. Higher levels increase the amount of fat available to burn off.

This benefit has been confirmed in research. In one study, researchers put eleven healthy, lean subjects on an eighty-four-hour fast and analyzed levels of glucose and norepinephrine. They found that fasting increased norepinephrine and reduced glucose—a situation that sets the stage for fat-burning and weight loss.

Another study put people on a seventy-two-hour fast. The researchers observed that the sympathetic nervous system (SNS) controlled key aspects of fat-burning through the release of norepinephrine. Also, the secretion of norepinephrine increased metabolic rate, which further initiated fat-burning.

With this knowledge, we no longer have to totally blame wrong diets or lack of physical activity for weight gain and obesity. Clearly, hormonal imbalances may be compromising your weight-loss efforts. If you have unexplained weight gain or just can't seem to lose weight, no matter what, an imbalance of certain hormones in your body may be the problem. But there is much you can do to reverse these problems—with intermittent fasting, diet, sleep, stress management, and other components of a hormonally healthy lifestyle.

To view the 21 references cited in this chapter,
please visit cynthiathurlow.com/references.

Chapter 4

. . . .

Restore Your Sex Hormones, Thyroid, and Melatonin

I remember meeting Joyce for the first time—a beautiful, raven-haired woman in her late forties who had come to see me because of alarming changes taking place in her body all at once. "I feel like I'm falling apart, not just physically but sexually, too," she told me, her voice trembling. "I get sweaty at night all the time, and I can't sleep. I'm gaining weight around my waist, which has never happened, and I don't feel desirable. Sexually, I'm just not 'feeling it' with my husband, so our sex life has really dropped off."

If you're like Joyce—and like I had been several years before—you know exactly what she was describing: a bundle of symptoms pointing to the ebb and flow of certain hormones that takes place in all of us as we go through life. As unpleasant as these changes are, they happen to all of us in varying degrees of intensity, and they can be managed, even resolved, with nutrition, lifestyle changes, and intermittent fasting.

To understand how, you must get to know a few other key hormones, how they work, and why they are so connected to how you feel and function in your life.

For perspective, there are more than two hundred hormones or hormonelike substances that course through our bodies—which is both amazing and mind-boggling. Among these are our sex hormones—most notably estrogen and progesterone—which support normal reproductive function and the menstrual cycle, and help determine our physical characteristics, such as skin texture, muscle tone, and body shape. Another sex hormone important to women is testosterone. It boosts libido, helping us feel sexy and sensual. It also helps create bone and muscle mass and offers many other benefits.

Through a series of chemical reactions, all three are produced from cholesterol, a waxy white fatty material found in all cells of the body. About 75 percent of the cholesterol in the body comes not from what we eat but is produced by the liver. The remaining 25 percent is supplied by our diet from foods such as animal protein and healthy fats. So when it comes to balancing your hormones naturally, eating enough fat is important. It helps enhance hormone production and maintain a healthy hormone profile.

In this chapter, we'll look at other hormones besides our sex hormones, like thyroid hormones, which have a huge impact on metabolism and our moods. They are sensitive to imbalances in insulin and stress hormones but can respond beautifully to lifestyle changes.

You'll find that I talk a lot about sleep. There is just no substitute for a good night's sleep. It is vital for hormonal health and rebalancing. You can't catch up on sleep, either. Once it's gone, it's gone.

Most of the time you spend intermittent fasting occurs overnight, when you are asleep and your body is repairing, detoxing, and producing growth hormone. Sleep greatly affects your health. It can be helped along by the hormone melatonin, discussed here, which sets your sleep-wake cycle and circadian rhythm.

With all of these hormones and others in balance, you can restore the same state of health and well-being you once enjoyed as a younger version of you. You'll find that when your hormones are back in tune—and supported by diet, fasting, and positive lifestyle changes—you'll feel vibrantly healthy no matter what your age.

Estrogen—the Trio of Female Hormones

Estrogen is the collective name for a trio of female hormones: estradiol, secreted from the ovaries during your reproductive years; estriol, produced during pregnancy; and estrone, found in women after menopause.

Estradiol (E2) is the form we have in the greatest quantity in our fertile, cycling years and is the most powerful. It is responsible for increasing your sex drive and moisturizing body tissues, such as your skin, eyes, lips, and vagina. Levels start their descent during perimenopause and fall off even more after menopause.

Estriol (E3) accounts for about 10 percent of our total estrogen but predominates during pregnancy, when it is produced by the placenta. It is detectable only during pregnancy.

Of the three estrogens, estrone (E1) is the dominant form during menopause. It also constitutes about 10 percent of our total estrogen and is created primarily in our fat cells, ovaries, and adrenal glands. It is a weaker form of estrogen compared to estradiol.

Importance

These naturally occurring estrogens are responsible for developing our sexual characteristics, regulating menstrual cycles, and maintaining normal cholesterol levels.

In balance, estrogen keeps our skin soft and supple, protects against cardiovascular disease, affects memory, and prevents inflammation. It impacts our weight, too, since estrogen is also produced in fat cells. One of the chief reasons we tend to gain weight after hysterectomies and during perimenopause and menopause is due to changes in estrogen levels.

Around midlife, other factors compound this estrogen-related weight gain. You tend to lose metabolically active muscle tissue (a condition called sarcopenia) and develop insulin resistance. These are among the reasons many women struggle with their weight as they get older.

Imbalances

I work with many women who have an imbalance of two key hormones: estrogen and progesterone—a more permanent state of hormonal imbalance known as "estrogen dominance." With it, a woman has excessive estrogen levels but has less progesterone to balance estrogen.

Symptoms of estrogen dominance can be similar to those of perimenopause, menopause, or even PMS. They include mood swings, irritability, decreased sex drive, worsening PMS symptoms, irregular periods, heavy periods, bloating, weight gain, anxiety, hair loss, trouble sleeping, fatigue, brain fog, memory problems, hot flashes and night sweats, and fertility issues.

Estrogen dominance occurs in two ways. The first is endogenously—inside the body. The body makes too much estrogen, and it is not properly eliminated or metabolized. The second is exogenously—outside the body—in which we are exposed to artificial estrogens in the environment called xenoestrogens, and they are not properly eliminated from the body.

Factors that can prompt high levels of endogenous estrogen include:

- A fiber-deficient diet. Because fiber helps food pass through the digestive system, a low-fiber diet can prevent excess estrogen from being properly excreted, leading to reabsorption.
- Stress. The secretion of cortisol increases under extreme stress. In order to produce sufficient levels of cortisol, the adrenal glands may suppress progesterone production, causing elevated estrogen levels.
- Alcohol use. Research has proven that circulating levels of estrogen are significantly higher in women who drink excessively. Plus, damage to the liver from alcohol abuse hinders estrogen excretion.
- Caffeine. Excessive caffeine intake has been shown to increase estrogen production and secretion.
- Impaired liver detoxification. Normally your liver packages up any excess estrogen and helps eliminate it through your bowels. But if you're dealing with infrequent bowel movements, constipation,

poor-quality nutrition, or gut dysbiosis (meaning there are imbalances in your microbiome), these estrogens can be recirculated in the body rather than excreted.

Part of that microbiome is the "estrobolome," a collection of friendly bacteria capable of metabolizing and getting rid of excess estrogen. These microbes produce an enzyme called beta-glucuronidase. When the estrobolome is in good working order, it makes just the right amount of beta-glucuronidase to keep estrogen in balance.

But if you suffer from any of the above conditions, especially dysbiosis, beta-glucuronidase may get too high or out of balance, and estrogen will not be properly metabolized and excreted. This can lead to estrogen dominance and potentially trigger the development of estrogen-related illnesses, such as endometriosis and breast cancer.

Exogenous estrogens—xenoestrogens—are foreign and destructive estrogens from our environment that have estrogen-like effects. They mimic our natural hormones and can then block or bind receptors, creating harmful imbalances. They're in everything from self-care products to pesticides to plastics to milk and meat from hormone-fed cows.

Exposure to xenoestrogens can lead to an imbalance in estrogen and progesterone and can predispose someone to develop estrogen dominance. Also, like many toxins, xenoestrogens are not biodegradable so they get lodged in our fat cells and can be very difficult to eliminate from the body. The accumulation has been linked to breast cancer, obesity, infertility, endometriosis, early puberty, miscarriages, and diabetes.

Intermittent Fasting and Estrogen

Normally, your body maintains an optimal balance of estrogen and does so in two ways—by producing just the right amounts of hormones and by eliminating excess hormones by processing and excreting them from the body. Intermittent fasting helps with much of this.

First, fasting supports the interplay of estrogen and growth hormone. The more estrogen we have circulating, the more growth hormone we produce. So, what does this really mean for us? Both estrogen and growth hormones fall off as we get older, especially after the age of forty. We need growth hormone to help with "estrogen signaling," the ability of your cells to receive estrogen and for optimal communication between the brain and ovaries. Fasting helps increase growth hormone, which in turn helps maintain optimal estrogen levels through proper signaling.

Second, with xenoestrogens everywhere in our environment, we're more susceptible than ever to estrogen dominance. Because intermittent fasting cleans house at the cellular level, it can hasten the removal of excess toxic estrogen from the body.

Third, fasting supports your microbiome, as I mentioned in chapter 1. With a healthy microbiome and a healthy estrobolome, your gut bacteria can better detoxify estrogen and remove it from the body. Specifically, intermittent fasting helps reset the estrobolome through periodic digestive rest, corrects dysbiosis, and aids in preventing and reversing estrogen-related conditions.

Fourth, one of the most remarkable functions of intermittent fasting and estrogen has to do with breast cancer. Balanced estrogen protects against breast cancer and can help prevent it from returning. A study of women who received treatment following breast cancer found that those who intermittent fasted saw a 70 percent reduction in the recurrence of their cancer!

Why is this? Scientists aren't sure, but it may be because intermittent fasting can optimize estrogen balance and protect against a cancer-promoting, toxic environment in cells, possibly by boosting autophagy.

Progesterone—a Key Female Hormone

Progesterone is a female hormone that plays a role in menstruation, pregnancy, and the formation of embryos. It is made in the ovaries and placenta up until menopause. After menopause, it is produced in the adrenal glands.

Importance

Progesterone performs many functions in the body that help you maintain good health. It balances estrogen, is responsible for breast development, helps regulate sleep and body temperature, assists in bone formation, maintains blood-sugar levels, and supports the efficiency of the thyroid. By helping your bladder function normally, progesterone also acts as a natural diuretic. It relaxes the muscles in your gut, too, so that your body can break down food into nutrients that are absorbed and used elsewhere in your body.

With progesterone in balance, you're likely to feel less irritable or anxious or and less prone to have mood swings. Progesterone has a calming effect on the brain. It does so by stimulating receptors for gamma-aminobutyric acid (GABA). GABA is a neurotransmitter that naturally calms the brain by interrupting the transmission of anxiety messages from nerve cell to nerve cell.

Imbalances

Progesterone declines at certain points in your life: when your menstrual cycles stop, as ovulation becomes less frequent in perimenopause, and when you reach menopause. Other factors can cause a progesterone deficiency: stress; taking antidepressants; a poorly functioning thyroid; a shortfall of vitamins A, B6, and C and the mineral zinc; and too much sugar in your diet.

The symptoms of declining progesterone are increased anxiety, mid-sleep wakening and sleep disturbances, shorter menstrual cycles, breast tenderness, night sweats and hot flashes, increased cramps and painful menstruation (dysmenorrhea), migraines, PMS, and weight gain.

Intermittent Fasting and Progesterone

Progesterone can be sensitive to intermittent fasting. If you are cycling— meaning that you are still having your monthly period— you must fast at certain times during your cycle, or you can deplete this hormone. For example, do not fast for five to seven days prior to your time of menstruation. (More on this in chapter 5.) Otherwise, fasting can help support and balance healthy levels of progesterone.

Testosterone—the Libido Hormone

One of our other primary sex hormones, testosterone, is a member of a class of hormones called androgens. Another androgen is DHEA, which I discuss below. Androgens are typically found in greater quantities in men, but they exist in women, too. We don't have as much testosterone as men have, but what we do have exerts some powerful effects in our bodies. Testosterone is produced in the adrenal glands and ovaries.

Importance

Testosterone triggers sexual desire in women and is thus important for keeping libido high. But it helps you in many other ways. Testosterone:

- Builds bone and prevents it from deteriorating
- Maintains muscle mass (so you burn fat)
- Keeps your energy levels high
- Helps maintain memory
- Increases your sense of emotional well-being, self-confidence, and motivation

For testosterone to perform all these wonderful functions, estradiol must be optimized. Without enough of this estrogen around, testosterone cannot attach to your brain receptors. Estrogen thus plays a role in how well testosterone works—so once again, it's an orchestra, with every player affecting every other.

Imbalances

Like many other hormones, testosterone peaks around the age of twenty-five, then gradually falls off. With menopause, the natural production of our testosterone declines by about half. A short supply of testosterone can make it difficult to build muscle, which is so critical to weight, blood-sugar control, and other metabolic actions. Declining testosterone can also lower your sex drive.

If you are insulin resistant, you might have too much testosterone, so overcoming insulin resistance can help bring this hormone back into balance. Stress impacts the production of DHEA, which affects testosterone levels, too.

Intermittent Fasting and Testosterone

You can naturally boost your testosterone levels, and intermittent fasting can help. Remember that intermittent fasting is an excellent way to help correct insulin resistance. So when you fast, you balance insulin and create metabolic flexibility—both of which help improve your testosterone levels.

Fasting boosts your testosterone levels in another way. In a study from the *Journal of Clinical Endocrinology and Metabolism*, intermittent fasting lowered levels of the hunger hormone leptin. This decrease triggered an immediate surge of testosterone.

So yes—with intermittent fasting, you have a great deal of control over your testosterone levels.

Boost Testosterone Naturally

To increase testosterone:

- Exercise, especially with strength training and HIIT
- Increase your protein intake
- Manage stress effectively
- Obtain an adequate intake of vitamin D through sunshine, food, and supplementation
- Get quality sleep
- Supplement with adaptogens—dietary supplements that help balance hormones, support immune function, and assist the body in recovering from both short-term and long-term stress
  (See chapter 7 for more information.)

Dehydroepiandrosterone (DHEA)—
the Longevity Hormone

DHEA is an androgen naturally produced by the adrenal glands, as well as by the central nervous system (brain and spinal cord). It is the most abundant hormone in your bloodstream.

Importance

DHEA isn't a sex hormone per se, but it a building block for eighteen hormones, including estrogen and testosterone. DHEA has a long and positive list of benefits. This hormone:

- Promotes lean muscle development
- Helps your body burn fat
- Supports bone growth
- Gives you glowing skin
- Improves memory
- Strengthens immunity
- Eases stress responses

Imbalances

Peak DHEA production is between the ages of twenty and twenty-five. After this, production steadily falls off by about 10 percent each year. You may feel the side effects of this decline by the time you hit your forties: vaginal and skin dryness; mood problems like anxiety or depression; poor sleep; weight gain; loss of your sex drive; brain fog; and greater vulnerability to age-related diseases, such as osteoporosis and heart disease.

With chronic stress and its resulting high cortisol, DHEA levels can plummet, and the more you risk insulin resistance and metabolic inflexibility. DHEA levels are also inversely associated with insulin levels, meaning that when DHEA is low, insulin is high, and vice versa.

Intermittent Fasting and DHEA

As with all hormones, a healthy lifestyle can help improve your DHEA levels. This includes intermittent fasting, which helps you better balance cortisol and insulin, with the net result of naturally boosting DHEA and improving metabolic flexibility.

DHEA, like so many other hormones, rises in response to a healthy diet, free of sugar and processed carbohydrates. A good example of this is found in one of the longest-lived societies in the world: the Okinawans in Japan. Even at age sixty-five and higher, they have more natural DHEA in their bodies than Americans of the same age! The reason has to do mostly with their natural diet and frequent calorie restriction (intermittent fasting is a form of calorie restriction). So yes, there's no question that we can counter aging by what we eat, how much we eat, and when we eat.

Other Key Hormones

Thyroid Hormones—the Metabolic Regulators

This butterfly-shaped gland sits low on the front of your neck and is a major player when it comes to hormonal health because it orchestrates all cellular functions, mainly metabolism.

Importance

The thyroid gland is your metabolic regulator. It produces two hormones—T4 (thyroxine) and T3 (triiodothyronine)—that carry out various regulating functions in your body. T4 can convert to T3 (the active form of thyroid hormone). Thyroid hormones:

- Support the function of mitochondria
- Regulate your metabolic rate and energy
- Control your weight
- Govern the metabolism of protein, fat, and carbohydrates

- Adjust your internal temperature
- Help with tissue repair and development—including your skin, hair, and nails
- Control blood flow and oxygen utilization
- Are involved in your menstrual cycle
- Regulate vitamin usage by the body
- Any imbalance of thyroid hormones can thus affect every metabolic function in your body.

Imbalances

Your thyroid and your adrenals work together for the healthy hormonal operation of your sex hormones. For a woman, this means a smooth-running menstrual cycle or transition.

At perimenopause and menopause, thyroid problems can develop due to hormone imbalances. There are thyroid receptors on your ovaries, and your thyroid gland has ovary receptors. Therefore, the loss of estrogen and testosterone from your ovaries at menopause can compromise thyroid function.

There are two common thyroid problems related to the production of thyroid hormones. One is hypothyroidism, or an underactive thyroid. It occurs when your thyroid can't produce enough hormone to keep the body going as it normally does. It is not uncommon for women in perimenopause and beyond to develop an underactive thyroid.

Most cases of hypothyroidism are related to an autoimmune disorder called Hashimoto's thyroiditis, in which the immune system attacks the thyroid, creating inflammation. This is eight times more common in women than men and generally is diagnosed between the ages of forty and sixty. In fact, 90 percent of all those diagnosed with hypothyroidism suffer from Hashimoto's.

Fortunately, this disease is reversible, as is non-autoimmune hypothyroidism. You can obtain significant improvements after identifying and treating suspected underlying causes such as food sensitivities, infections, nutrient deficiencies, and toxins.

The other thyroid problem is hyperthyroidism, or an overactive thyroid. In this case, the thyroid gland produces too much hormone. This is called Grave's disease and is less common, impacting 2 to 3 percent of the general population.

Grave's disease is an autoimmune disease, too, and is characterized by the abnormal enlargement of the thyroid (goiter) and increased secretion of thyroid hormone. Once you're diagnosed and start treatment, including medication and diet, this, too, can be improved, stabilized, or even reversed.

Intermittent Fasting and the Thyroid

Thyroid disorders come with a host of problems like weight issues, brain fog, and fatigue. On the bright side, intermittent fasting can help resolve these issues for many thyroid patients. It can definitely help people lose weight. By lowering insulin and promoting metabolic flexibility, it reduces inflammation. This is important because in Hashimoto's and Grave's disease, especially, the thyroid can be chronically inflamed. By enhancing mitochondrial health, intermittent fasting eases brain fog and fights fatigue.

I am frequently asked if those with a thyroid diagnosis can safely intermittent fast. I truly believe that this is bio-individual, meaning that it will be specific to the person who is considering fasting.

As I noted, fasting is a hormetic stressor. In order for fasting to work for you, many factors must align properly. Your sleep quality must be excellent. You must deal with stress proactively. Your medications should be successfully managing your symptoms. And you should be consuming a nutrient-dense, whole-foods diet.

Even so, some studies and experts advise being careful with fasting. One study looked at thyroid function in obese people who fasted for four days. (They did not have any preexisting thyroid issues.) The fast depressed their thyroid function. It went back to normal after they started eating mixed meals that included carbohydrates, protein, and fats.

Another study looked again at Ramadan fasting. During the fast, people of the Muslim faith abstain from both food and drink, even water, until sunset. In healthy Muslim women, Ramadan fasting triggered drops in T4 and T3 during the last few days of Ramadan.

The reason for these side effects is most likely due to the fact that while fasting, you're not taking in any calories. This sends a message to the body that "times are tough." The thyroid answers the message by slowing your metabolism and preserving energy and nutrients. So I would advise, if you are being treated for thyroid disease, please be cautious and work closely with your health care provider.

But, let's be clear, I myself have an underactive thyroid, as do many of my patients and clients. We can successfully fast, as long as other healthy lifestyle measures are in place.

Melatonin—the Sleep/Wake Hormone

I'd like to finish this chapter with a discussion of melatonin because it has a relationship with many of the hormones we've covered. Melatonin is secreted by the pineal gland, located in the middle of the brain called the suprachiasmatic nucleus, or SCN. Its job is to set and regulate the internal clock that controls your circadian rhythm. Its production increases with evening darkness and it promotes deep, healthy sleep.

Importance

Melatonin influences your body in many ways—beyond helping you sleep and monitoring your internal clock. Melatonin:

- Affects the release of your sex hormones
- Boosts your immune system
- Acts as an antioxidant to help prevent disease
- Decreases cortisol and helps balance your stress response
- Stimulates the production of growth hormone
- Regulates the synthesis of testosterone
- Improves mood

Imbalances

Like all hormones, melatonin does not work in isolation. It interacts with other hormones to regulate your internal environment and overall health.

Melatonin has a lot in common with insulin, for example. The pancreas, which releases insulin, is very sensitive to melatonin levels. Melatonin levels rise during nighttime hours, while insulin levels are at their lowest. Melatonin actually slows insulin production while you're asleep. This makes sense when you think about the role of insulin. When you're asleep, your energy needs are low. Because you aren't eating or digesting food while asleep, your body doesn't require peak levels of insulin to deal with rising blood sugar. And, because you're in a period of fasting during sleep, low levels of insulin at night actually stabilize blood-sugar levels, preventing hypoglycemia, until you eat again the next day.

But if melatonin levels are low, insulin activity is not suppressed at night. This means your pancreas doesn't get its nightly break from making insulin. With insulin levels elevated around the clock, your pancreas can become inefficient at making enough insulin, or the cells in your body can become desensitized to too much insulin. This can lead to insulin resistance.

Melatonin also has a relationship with estrogen. Estrogen is required to produce serotonin, known as the "happy neurotransmitter" because of its positive effect on mood. During menopause, there is a decline in estrogen, resulting in low serotonin levels. To make matters worse, reduced serotonin levels lead to low melatonin levels. This is because serotonin is involved in manufacturing melatonin.

This crazy imbalance of melatonin, estrogen, serotonin, and insulin creates the perfect storm for menopausal symptoms like mood swings and sleep disorders. Fortunately, both serotonin and melatonin levels can be boosted through dietary changes and nutritional supplements.

Melatonin is also influenced by cortisol. In fact, they are agonists and fight for dominance in the body. Normally, melatonin takes control at night, slowing down production of cortisol and encouraging proper rest and repair overnight. In the morning, melatonin wanes and cortisol and other adrenal hormones take over, making you alert and giving you energy. But if you're struggling with chronic stress, this cycle doesn't shut down properly. Cortisol stays high at night and melatonin production is inadequate. You can't sleep and end up feeling worn out all the time.

Also, if your melatonin levels are low and your quality of sleep is poor, this directly affects how much growth hormone your body makes. Not good, either! Remember, growth hormone is an age eraser. It is released during sleep, so if you're not sleeping well, aging can accelerate.

Exposure to blue light from computers, cell phones, or television screens prior to bedtime can interfere with the secretion of melatonin and increase cortisol instead, keeping you awake. Additionally, not getting enough sunlight, especially first thing in the morning, can further jeopardize proper secretion of melatonin and cortisol. Just five to ten minutes of light exposure in the morning can make a huge difference in your day.

Intermittent Fasting and Melatonin

I never had much trouble with my sleep until I entered my forties. I spent more time awake in bed, and it took me longer to fall asleep. And sometimes, I didn't even sleep through the night. Everyone has an occasional sleepless night—because of worry, anxiety, excitement, or jet lag. But those are different from my situation—chronic sleeplessness and the inability to get the rest my body needed.

Then I began to incorporate intermittent fasting into my life. I was amazed by what happened. Over time, I started sleeping soundly through the night—a result of balancing melatonin, insulin, estrogen, and serotonin through not only intermittent fasting but also through changes I made to my nutrition, to my exercise program, and to the way I was handling stress. It all works together in a rather wonderful fashion to balance hormones involved in promoting sleep quality. I can't wait to tell you more about all of this when we get to Part 2, which covers the intermittent fasting lifestyle.

So there you have it—a view into other incredible hormones and how intermittent fasting affects each one. As we get older, they fluctuate quite a bit. Aging means that we produce more of some hormones and less of others. But with a little age also comes a little wisdom, and learning how to balance your hormones with intermittent fasting and other strategies will improve the quality of your life, and perhaps even extend it.

To view the 17 references cited in this chapter,
please visit cynthiathurlow.com/references.

Chapter 5

. . . .

Intermittent Fasting
and Your Life Stage

Many fasting programs ignore how beautifully unique we are as women. Our uniqueness is attributable to many things, but it is definitely impacted by how our hormones change from day to day and hour by hour for most of our lives. They affect how we think, how we communicate, and how we navigate our way of being in the world.

In addition, our bodies are very different from men's in other ways—in our ability to conceive a child and give birth, and in the distinct nature of our transition through various life stages.

As a woman, you are likely to live five years longer than a man. But you're also at risk for various health problems: breast cancer, alcohol abuse, heart disease and stroke, osteoporosis, osteoarthritis, depression and anxiety, stress, sexually transmitted diseases, and urinary tract infections. Many of these conditions become more common after you stop menstruating and begin your journey toward menopause, when there are changes in your hormones.

The female brain is smaller than a male's, but on the plus side, our brains are approximately four years younger than men's, at least in how they burn fuel, according to scans performed by researchers at Washington University School of Medicine in St. Louis. This may help explain why we tend to stay mentally sharp for longer.

We feel conflict more deeply, we report more work stress, tension, and frustration than men, and we often respond by working harder. We empathize more, can feel what others feel, and are highly caring and protective of our loved ones. We are pretty amazing.

All these attributes make us more sensitive than men to environmental, nutritional, and lifestyle changes and cues. And they all dictate what diet, fasting plan, exercise program, supplements, and more that work best for our bodies. There is simply no one-size-fits-all plan for women—which is why I will teach you how to set up an intermittent fasting plan based, first and foremost, on whether you are cycling, in perimenopause, or in menopause (and beyond). Each stage requires a unique approach to fasting and nutrition.

The Infradian Rhythm and Cycling

When you're cycling, your body goes through adjustments as your hormone levels fluctuate throughout the month. Your metabolism changes, as do cortisol levels, which can affect your response to stress. You require a different amount of sleep, may feel more tired throughout the day, and perhaps battle premenstrual syndrome (PMS) from time to time.

Each of these things is due to your unique "infradian rhythm," otherwise known as your internal menstrual clock. Similar to the circadian rhythm, which covers twenty-four hours, our infradian rhythm occurs over our twenty-eight-day menstrual cycle. Every woman who is menstruating has an infradian rhythm, and it helps to regulate your cycle.

Over the course of a twenty-eight-day infradian rhythm, you move through three distinct phases, ending in menstruation:

Phase 1: Follicular
Phase 2: Ovulatory
Phase 3: Luteal

During each phase, your body shifts its energy levels, temperature, metabolism, glucose ups and downs, cortisol levels, sleep quality, and so forth. You may notice, for example, that you sleep better during certain phases of your cycle over others or your skin glows more.

Also, your metabolism speeds up and slows down predictably across the month. This is why you need to change what you eat, do intermittent fasting, and increase intensity of your workouts each week. All of these actions optimize your metabolism.

You need more sleep than men because as a woman, you have a more complex brain and it needs more time to restore itself and reset cognitively for the next day.

If you are still cycling, supporting your infradian rhythm is important so that you feel your best and perform at your best, even as your hormones act wildly. Support comes in the form of intermittent fasting, nutrition, movement, and other lifestyle factors.

The Phases of Cycling

From the time of your first period—around the age of twelve—until menopause at about age fifty-one or fifty-two—you can count on three to seven days of bleeding every month or so—referred to as menstruation. Over the years, the duration of bleeding shortens, with longer stretches between periods. You may be one of many women who has menstrual difficulties, such as PMS, a collection of symptoms—bloating, painful cramps, breast tenderness, headaches, moodiness, irritability, weight gain, cravings, and more.

Cycling is more than just a period. It is the culmination of a hormonal cycle involving the follicular, ovulatory, and luteal phases. The end result is menstruation, in which you bleed as your uterus sheds its lining. It occurs on days 1 through 5 of your cycle. Here is a closer look at each phase.

Follicular

As you begin your menstrual cycle, your body prepares itself to receive a fertilized egg for implantation in the uterus. In this phase, estrogen levels are low but steadily increase to prepare for ovulation (the release of an egg) and potential pregnancy.

Rising estrogen increases levels of luteinizing hormone (LH), which controls the function of your ovaries. A decrease in estrogen triggers the release of follicle-stimulating hormone (FSH). This hormone encourages your ovaries to create several small sacs called follicles, from which estrogen is produced. Each follicle contains an immature egg. The healthiest egg matures while the rest of the follicles get reabsorbed into the body. At this point, your body begins to release extra estrogen. The follicular phase typically covers days 6 to 14 of your cycle. It ends when you ovulate.

During the follicular phase, there is a delicate balance between too much and too little estrogen—an imbalance that can be good and bad. This can cause, for example:

- A slower metabolism
- Lower cortisol
- Higher energy levels
- Good moods

If estrogen is higher and more dominant, glucose levels tend to be lower during the follicular phase. Your cells thus tend to be more insulin-sensitive at this time, because estrogen actually helps your body use insulin more normally.

In upcoming chapters, I cover specific foods to eat in your feeding window, as well as how to exercise, but I want to explain here how to eat in sync with your cycle, as well as how to exercise.

To support yourself nutritionally during the follicular phase:

- Eat foods high in zinc, namely seafood, and most notably oysters. Zinc has many functions in the body, but it mostly supports and revives your immune function. It is also an antioxidant mineral, capable of fighting off molecules called free radicals that roam your body, attacking cells and promoting aging.
- Focus on phytoestrogen-containing foods that support healthy estrogen levels in the body. These include chickpeas, peanuts, flaxseeds, grapes, berries, plums, green and black tea, and others.
- Eat fermented foods like kimchi and high-quality fermented vegetables like cabbage, carrots, cauliflower, garlic, cucumbers, or even

low-sugar kombucha (5 grams of sugar or less per serving). These foods can help build a diverse microbiome.

- Be sure to get enough omega-3 fatty acids, mostly from fatty fish. Among many other benefits, these fats fight inflammation in the body and help balance the inflammatory omega-6 fatty acids that are so widespread in the diets of most Westernized adults.
- Enjoy lighter meals, with non-starchy vegetables, such as salad veggies, broccoli, cauliflower, Brussels sprouts, green leafy vegetables, among others; and non-processed starches such as sweet potatoes, winter squash, or legumes. I can't say enough about vegetables. They contain nutrients that build health, prevent disease, and pretty much put aging on hold.

As for physical activity, concentrate on:

- Cardio exercise and high-intensity interval training (HIIT)
- Hiking, running, or jogging
- Strength training with heavier weights
- Cross-training

Ovulatory

This phase begins when the ovary releases a mature egg for a potential pregnancy. Covering days 15 to 17 of your cycle, ovulation is marked by peaks in estrogen, progesterone, and testosterone.

During ovulation, the egg leaves the ovary, travels down the fallopian tube, and makes its way to the uterus. At any time during this journey, sperm can fertilize the egg. It can survive for about twenty-four hours before it needs to be fertilized.

During the ovulatory phase, expect to feel:

- A higher sex drive
- More confidence
- Higher energy levels

To support yourself nutritionally during the ovulatory phase:

- Focus on foods rich in vitamin C (fruits, broccoli, and leafy greens). Vitamin C helps you deal with physical and emotional stress—which in turn lowers levels of stress hormones. This vitamin also stops skin from sagging by boosting collagen. Collagen is one of the structural proteins in the body that supports skin, soft tissue, and joints.
- Include foods high in B vitamins (grass-fed and organic animal proteins and gluten-free whole grains). The B vitamins play important roles in energy production and help calm and maintain a healthy nervous system.
- Eat phytonutrient-rich fruits and vegetables, including fresh herbs and spices. Phytonutrients help prevent illness and have a positive influence on hormone balance.
- Fill your plate with cruciferous vegetables (broccoli, cabbage, cauliflower, Brussels sprouts, and so forth). They contain natural chemicals that speed the removal of harmful and excess estrogens from the body.
- Have healthy fats (olive oil, coconut oil, avocados, nuts, and seeds, among others). Ovulation is an energy-demanding phase, so we need these fats, as well as omega-3 fatty acids for pregnancy, nursing, energy, hormone production, and brain health.
- Emphasize quality, grass-fed, and organic protein at meals. Adequate protein ensures that your body can build, repair, and maintain your muscles, connective tissue, skin, and organs. It is also important for satiety.
- Include foods that support your liver health. For proper detoxification, your liver loves garlic; beets; fruits such as grapes, plums, and grapefruit; fermented foods; cruciferous vegetables; dandelion greens; asparagus; artichokes; and green tea.

As for physical activity, concentrate on activities that support your higher energy levels:

- Sprinting and high-intensity interval training (HIIT)
- Running, or jogging
- Spinning
- Circuit training

Luteal Phase

Triggered by sudden drops in estrogen, FSH, and LH, the luteal phase covers days 18 to 28 of your cycle. The follicle morphs into a mass of cells called the corpus luteum. The corpus luteum secretes large amounts of progesterone. The hormone is responsible for thickening the uterine lining into a plush, nutritive bed in which a fertilized egg may implant and develop into an embryo.

If the egg is not fertilized, the corpus luteum dissolves into the body. Both estrogen and progesterone levels drop abruptly. The egg will dissolve, too, and the uterine lining sloughs off in the form of menstrual flow. This end result is referred to as menstruation—those one to five days of your cycle, referred to as your period.

If estrogen and progesterone get out of balance during this phase, PMS symptoms can develop.

During the ovulatory phase, expect to:

- Feel hungrier as your energy intake increases
- Have more food cravings
- Have lower energy levels
- Be moody

Your glucose levels tend to rise during the luteal phase. This elevation can reduce insulin sensitivity, which means that insulin is doing a poor job of moving glucose into cells for energy, leading to higher circulating glucose. You're thus more prone to insulin resistance during your luteal phase.

To support yourself nutritionally and to avoid PMS during the luteal phase:

- Because your body is more insulin resistant during the luteal phase, avoid carb-heavy or sugary foods and prioritize low-carb foods such as green leafy vegetables, cruciferous vegetables, and salad veggies for optimal metabolic health. Also, stay away from alcohol, added sugars, dairy, and processed foods (which promote insulin resistance and sugar cravings).
- Focus on minerals: magnesium-rich foods (dark chocolate, nuts, seeds, and spinach) and selenium-rich foods (Brazil nuts). But watch excess sodium (salt) intake to prevent bloating.
- Include omega-3 fatty acids from fatty fish and other healthy fats.
- Concentrate on foods high in B vitamins.
- Support your digestion with fiber-rich vegetables such as dark leafy greens and unprocessed gluten-free starches.

Your stamina may be low during this phase, so concentrate on the following activities:

- Light to moderate exercise
- Strength training
- Pilates
- Yoga
- Low-intensity cardio (such as walking)

Menstruation
This is the time in which the lining of your uterus sheds, creating bleeding. Estrogen and progesterone are both low, and your energy levels and mood may be low, too.

To support yourself nutritionally during the menstruation phase:

- Concentrate on foods high in B vitamins.
- Focus on magnesium-rich foods (dark chocolate, nuts, seeds, and spinach)
- Include omega-3 fatty acids from fatty fish.

- Eat colorful fruits and vegetables. These foods are high in phytonutrients and antioxidants, which are nutrients that help protect the body from free radical damage. Colorful plant foods are rich in pain-killing, inflammation-reducing pigments, and because each color of a vegetable provides a different pigment, the more variety you eat, the more health benefits you get.
- Add beets and medicinal mushrooms to your meals. Beets are good for your circulatory system, which supports energy levels by oxygenating the body and transporting nutrients through the blood to tissues and organs. They also protect the gallbladder, helping it break down and emulsify fats. Mushrooms like the shiitake variety deserve more nutritional credit than they've received. They are very powerful inflammation fighters.
- Drink bone broth and herbal teas. Bone broth supplies collagen, an important protein for skin and joint health, and minerals. Certain herbal teas help relieve PMS symptoms: chasteberry, dandelion, red raspberry leaf, and chamomile, among others.
- Eat unprocessed gluten-free starches such as brown rice, sweet potatoes, and legumes.
- Emphasize quality, grass-fed, and organic protein at meals.
- Stay away from alcohol, caffeine, excess salt, and greasy and fatty foods.

As for physical activity, concentrate on gentle activities, punctuated by rest, that support your lower energy levels:

- Light and low movement
- Restorative yoga
- Stretching
- Meditation
- Connecting with nature

Intermittent Fasting During Cycling

If you are cycling, you may be wondering how you can support and optimize your menstrual cycle naturally. You may be curious to learn if fasting is even healthy for you. You may also want to know, through natural means, how to reduce PMS symptoms and other symptoms related to your menstrual cycle.

Most women I work with have the same questions. The answer is yes. You can do intermittent fasting as long as you pay attention to hormone fluctuations that occur over your twenty-eight-day cycle and focus on the best foods that can support your menstrual cycle.

Here are key guidelines:

1. If you are age thirty-five or under, adopt a flexible fasting schedule, such as every other day or a few days a week, so that you don't risk the possibility of throwing off your menstrual cycle. This approach is in contrast to a more regular fasting schedule that can be followed by a woman north of forty and closer to perimenopause and menopause.

2. I generally advise women not to fast if they are planning on becoming pregnant. Women need a good supply of energy and nutrients, obtained from food and stored as fat, in order to support a healthy pregnancy. When the female body does not get enough quality food and undergoes other stressors like lack of sleep, reproduction and fertility can potentially be impacted. You could also lose your period temporarily, a condition called amenorrhea.

3. With intermittent fasting, the first three weeks of your cycle are the best times to fast if you have a twenty-eight-day cycle. This is the time in which your hormones are more stable, and it is a great time to decrease insulin, reduce inflammation, and activate autophagy. However, fasting during the five to seven days preceding your menstrual cycle may unknowingly lead to the depletion of nutrients and hormones necessary in the luteal phase.

4.   Fasting is beneficial in specific circumstances. For example, women with PCOS would likely benefit from a fasting strategy, especially if they have weight to lose. A schedule of fasting for 12 to 16 hours, dependent on each individual, may help balance hormones, including insulin, and support weight loss. You have to be careful here, though, and not proceed if you are trying to conceive.

5.   Tune in to your stress levels. If you're under a lot of stress, postpone fasting until your situation becomes more manageable. Remember, when you fast, cortisol goes up, which can lead to imbalances in both estrogen and progesterone. It can even lead to a loss of your period. Not getting your period is a sign that your body is under too much stress to fast! To manage stress proactively, see my recommendations on pages 143–147.

6.   Get plenty of nutrients during your feeding window—and at other times when you are not fasting. Do not focus on calorie restriction.

Also, if intermittent fasting creates nutrient deficiencies or triggers prolonged low blood sugar (hypoglycemia), this will likely impact the hypothalamus-pituitary-adrenal axis and disrupt the production of reproductive hormones. In general, if you can't properly regulate your blood sugar, it is a sign that fasting may not be the right strategy for you. For many women, I start with ensuring that each meal is focused on protein and healthy fats. Once their blood sugar is better stabilized, they can start intermittent fasting.

Refer to the meal plans on pages 214–222. They make it easy for you to fast safely—and with very positive, hormone-balancing benefits.

Perimenopause

Perimenopause is a unique time in our lives, in which our sex hormones begin to wax and wane. This period has been virtually ignored in most medical research, yet it is a time of profound hormonal and physiological change. No longer do our bodies release an egg each month during ovulation, and our cycles become more irregular due to a decline in progesterone.

Other hormones ebb and flow. Cortisol levels tend to rise, worsening our stress response and disrupting other hormones. We're also more prone to insulin resistance. Less melatonin is secreted, so getting a good night's sleep is a challenge.

Estrogen is one hormone very much affected during perimenopause. For one thing, levels of estrogen, particularly estradiol, tend to rise at the start of perimenopause and this is a direct response to lowered levels of circulating progesterone. During this life stage, there's a sort of seesaw between estrogen and progesterone—when one hormone increases, the other will decrease.

A statistical review of studies found that during the follicular phase, estradiol levels were 30 percent higher in perimenopausal women than in women who were cycling. But toward the end of perimenopause, estradiol starts to decline.

The chief hallmarks of perimenopause are the increasing variability in the length of your menstrual cycle, the frequency of ovulation, and levels of reproductive hormones. Not much is known about why this variability occurs. But some evidence suggests that the dwindling pool of follicles itself is responsible. Another hypothesis is that the hypothalamus loses its ability to regulate menstrual cycles.

For some women, the symptoms of perimenopause may be rockier than going through menopause. But it doesn't have to be this way! Intermittent fasting can definitely help.

Common perimenopausal symptoms include irregular menstruation and ovulation cycles; hot flashes, night sweats, and sleep problems; mood changes; vaginal and bladder problems; changes in libido; loss of bone; and cardiovascular factors.

Irregular Menstruation and Ovulation Cycles

As you get a little older, so do your ovaries. We are born with a finite number of eggs, unlike men, who produce and replenish new sperm every three days. Aging leads to the erratic release of eggs during the ovulatory phase. This disruption depletes progesterone levels and interferes with the regularity of your cycle.

Your bleeding may be heavy, and one reason is related to estrogen dominance. Heavy bleeding can lead to anemia, dizziness, or worsening PMS, among other symptoms. As ovulation turns more unpredictable, the length of time between your periods may be longer or shorter, your flow may even get lighter, and you may skip some periods.

Hot Flashes, Night Sweats, and Sleep Problems

Hot flashes and night sweats are common during perimenopause, generally because the hypothalamus is not accustomed to falling estrogen levels. The intensity, length, and frequency of hot flashes and night sweats vary. They can be caused by low estradiol, blood-sugar fluctuations, food sensitivities, and gut problems. Night sweats and hot flashes occur in up to 60 percent of all perimenopausal women.

Hot flashes and night sweats disrupt sleep. But even if you don't have them, perimenopause can still be a time of sleepless nights. One reason has to do with variability in the secretion of melatonin, which helps you sleep. On pages 140–143, I cover guidelines to support proper melatonin production at night.

Mood Changes

If you find yourself in perimenopause and your mood swings are more intense, you are not alone. For a variety of reasons, women in this life stage feel more irritable, anxious, and depressed than when they were younger. The causes are largely hormonal, but poor sleep and life stresses—like job demands, taking care of older parents, changes in health, and so forth—can worsen your mood. If you are concerned, even if you're going through a tough time, you should absolutely seek professional help and counseling. What you are feeling is very real.

Vaginal and Bladder Problems

When estrogen levels diminish (usually toward the end of perimenopause), vaginal tissues become dry and lose lubrication. This makes intercourse

potentially painful. Low estrogen may make you more susceptible to urinary tract or vaginal infections. Loss of bladder tissue tone may lead to
urinary incontinence, which, though not fun, is treatable and reversible.

Changes in Libido
During perimenopause, you may begin to lose your desire for sex and feel
less aroused. But if you had satisfactory sexual intimacy prior to perimenopause, your libido may not be affected.

Loss of Bone
Your risk of osteoporosis—a disease that causes fragile bones—rises after
perimenopause, due mostly to declining estrogen. You gradually start to
lose bone more quickly than your body can replace it. Nutritional and
lifestyle habits help prevent osteoporosis: eating calcium-rich foods (broccoli, collard greens, fatty fish such as salmon and sardines); limiting alcohol use; not smoking; strength training; and maintaining adequate vitamin
D levels.

Cardiovascular Factors
Estrogen is important to your cardiovascular system because it keeps your
arteries flexible. But during perimenopause, your risk of developing heart
disease begins to rise. One factor is declining estrogen toward the end of
perimenopause and throughout menopause.

Intermittent fasting has been shown to alleviate major risk factors of
heart disease, including insulin resistance, metabolic inflexibility, inflammation, and high blood pressure. It also triggers cells to fight inflammation, and inflammation can lead to the buildup of arterial plaques that
cause heart attacks and stroke. People who incorporate fasting into their
lifestyles were 70 percent less likely to suffer heart failure than those who
had never fasted, according to a 2019 study in *Circulation*.

The Perimenopausal Timeline
Fortunately, these changes don't all come at once! Nor do they affect all
women. Nor is perimenopause one continuous process, as previously

thought. It has now been proposed as having five distinct phases, each with its own symptoms. In the earliest phases of perimenopause, you may not even perceive the subtle signs. However, as you progress through each phase, your symptoms become more noticeable. One of these is weight gain, caused by fluctuating estrogen, which occurs in the early part of perimenopause. Your body starts looking around for additional estrogen and finds it in your fat stores, which produces estrone. The result of finding this estrogen "replacement" is that your body begins to deposit more fat, especially around your midsection.

When you know the signs, you can begin to give your body even more intelligent care, including a smart diet and exercise program, and you can overcome many of these symptoms. The chart below walks you through each phase and lists the symptoms and the hormonal changes that occur over time.

Note that perimenopause ends when one full year has elapsed without menstruation. The average age of perimenopause is forty-seven and a half years, although no woman is average. If you're a smoker or have not ever had children, it may begin at an earlier age.

The Five Phases of Perimenopause and Their Symptoms

	PHASE A	PHASE B	PHASE C	PHASE D	PHASE E
Duration	2–6 months	2–6 months	1–2 years	1–2 years	1 year
Menstrual Cycles	Regular and ovulatory cycles	Regular cycles, but a shortened luteal phase; no egg is released	Alternating short and skipped cycles	Menstrual periods are infrequent; ovulation occurs 50 percent of the time	Menstrual cycle ceases
Flow	Abnormally heavy flow	Abnormally heavy flow	Unpredictable flow	Light, unpredictable flow; spotting may alternate with flooding	None

	PHASE A	PHASE B	PHASE C	PHASE D	PHASE E
Duration	2–6 months	2–6 months	1–2 years	1–2 years	1 year
Symptoms	Breast tenderness, mood swings, fluid retention, PMS symptoms, early morning night sweats, weight gain, migraines	PMS symptoms increase, menstrual cramps	Increased night sweats; hot flashes more common	Hot flashes and increased night sweats; some women may experience cramping	Hot flashes and night sweats may persist, but other perimenopausal symptoms begin to decrease: no more PMS, no more cramps, less breast tenderness, and fewer mood swings
Hormonal changes	Estrogen is fluctuating. FSH and LH are still normal; a hormone called inhibin— which is involved in the development of reproductive organs, fertility, and pregnancy— is low	FSH is intermittently elevated during the follicular phase, LH is normal, and estradiol is high.	FSH is still elevated, LH is occasionally elevated, and estradiol is high but may fluctuate.	Low progesterone levels; FSH and LH are persistently elevated; estradiol may be intermittently high or low.	FSH and LH are still high; estradiol may decline or may normalize.

Source: https://academic.oup.com/edrv/article/19/4/397/2530801.

Estrogen Dominance During Perimenopause

The level of estrogen in your body rises and falls unevenly during peri-menopause. At the beginning of perimenopause, estrogen levels rise. This coincides with declining progesterone and can lead to estrogen domi-nance.

Estrogen dominance can occur throughout your lifetime but is particularly problematic during perimenopause and is a major underlying factor of many perimenopause symptoms. To minimize estrogen dominance:

- Reduce your exposure to toxic xenoestrogens from self-care products, plastic containers, nonorganic foods, and other sources.
- Eat more cruciferous veggies. They have high levels of a natural compound called I3C (indole-3-carbinol). It helps detoxify excess estrogen in the liver.
- Support your liver health. The liver filters your blood so that it can be free of excess hormones and toxins. You can enhance your liver and its detoxification function by eating anti-inflammatory foods (refer to the next chapter), and including the liver-support foods I listed on page 69.
- Avoid or limit alcohol and stay away from recreational and illegal drugs. All of these substances are highly damaging to your liver.
- Practice intermittent fasting to help detox your body from excess estrogen.

Intermittent Fasting During Perimenopause

Perimenopause and intermittent fasting can be a beautiful relationship, but the trick is to ensure that you can successfully integrate fasting into a lifestyle that is balanced with sleep quality, effective stress management, healthy nutrition, and other lifestyle modifications. Intermittent fasting won't work otherwise, especially at this stage in your life.

Additionally, if you are still cycling, follow the same guidelines I listed for cycling women. Remember, with intermittent fasting, the first twenty-one days of your cycle are the best times to fast if you have a twenty-eight-day cycle, for the reasons mentioned earlier.

Pay attention to your stress levels. If you're under a lot of stress, postpone fasting until your situation becomes more manageable. Remember, when you fast, cortisol goes up, which lowers progesterone and increases estrogen. If you're in phase E of perimenopause, however, and you fast while under stress, estrogen can get depleted instead.

For stress reduction, see my suggestions on pages 143–147. Also, refer to the specific fasting and feeding meal plans for women on pages 214–222.

Menopause and Beyond

The medical definition of menopause is the complete cessation of menstrual periods for twelve consecutive months. The average age is fifty-one.

Around 15 percent of women who experience menopause say they went through it with no discomfort at all. Others are not so fortunate, since at menopause, a woman undergoes further hormonal upheaval. There is a dramatic decline in estrogen, progesterone, and testosterone, for example. This results in other symptoms, including many that you experienced during perimenopause:

- Hot flashes and night sweats
- Susceptibility to bladder infections (the thinning of the vaginal wall affects the bladder)
- Flatulence and bloating—often a result of dysbiosis
- Joint and muscle pain
- Osteoporosis
- Vaginal dryness and pain during intercourse
- Brain fog, with diminished concentration and short-term memory
- Headaches and migraines
- Mild depression and mood swings

What you require from your diet as a menopausal woman changes with your age. For example, during and after menopause:

- Increase your hydration with minerals called electrolytes (this is appropriate for all age ranges!). Drink half your body weight in ounces of water daily, supplemented with electrolytes. This can help relieve vaginal dryness caused by declining estrogen and the loss of connective tissue such as collagen and elastin. Proper hydration also relieves bloating. For information on electrolytes, see chapter 7.

- Concentrate on high-quality proteins. The decline in estrogen from menopause is linked to decreased muscle mass (sarcopenia) and decreased bone strength (osteopenia). For this reason, women going through menopause should eat protein, particularly grass-fed and organic, to avoid xenoestrogenic toxins.

- Emphasize strength training in your exercise routine. Lifting weights or performing any type of resistance training—with resistance bands or even your own body weight—also prevents sarcopenia and osteopenia.

- Continue to eat healthy fats, such as olive oil, coconut oil, avocados, nuts and seeds, nut butters, and others. Fats from these foods support hormonal balance. Omega-3 fatty acids from fish can decrease the frequency of hot flashes and the severity of night sweats, plus provide an excellent source of anti-inflammatory nutrition. These fats are delicious and easy to overeat, so just watch your portions, because they are a calorie-dense food.

- Boost calcium. A very important mineral for menopausal women is calcium. Your calcium needs increase during menopause because the loss of estrogen can speed up bone loss. It's best to get calcium from food but not dairy products because dairy products can be highly allergenic and inflammatory. Aim to get calcium from non-dairy sources such as sardines, kale, collard greens, turnip greens, beet greens, mustard greens, spinach, bok choy, almonds, chia seeds, sesame seeds, and other calcium-rich plant foods.

- Get enough vitamin D. This vitamin should already be a part of your daily routine, but right now, it is critical for protecting your bones during menopause. Vitamin D comes from the sun, but you can get it from certain foods like fatty fish and mushrooms. Plus, it's vital to supplement with this vitamin. It's on my A-list for women during menopause because research has linked it to preventing heart disease, osteoporosis, diabetes, cancer, and weight gain. Talk to your health care provider about the right amount for you.

- Increase fruits and vegetables. By filling up on these foods, you can help minimize weight gain while getting the nutrients and fiber you need to stay healthy. In a one-year intervention study in more than seventeen thousand menopausal women, those eating more vegetables, fruit, and fiber experienced a 19 percent reduction in hot flashes compared to the control group. Cruciferous vegetables are of supreme importance for menopausal and postmenopausal women. In another study, eating broccoli decreased levels of a type of estrogen linked to breast cancer, while increasing levels of an estrogen type that protects against breast cancer.

- All fruits are packed with antioxidant power and can possibly save you from many diseases. Berries in particular—blueberries, raspberries, strawberries, cranberries, and so forth—contain many health-promoting chemicals. They all are a good source of vitamin C, which boosts brain function and mood. Cranberries protect against urinary tract infections, which is a symptom after menopause in some women. I advise women to consume vegetables to fruits in a 3:1 ratio, so prioritize non-starchy vegetables over fruit.

- Have some gluten-free whole grains in small portions, if you tolerate them. Some ancient whole grains, such as millet, amaranth, teff, buckwheat, or even quinoa (which is actually a seed) or brown rice provide B vitamins—which help boost energy, manage stress, and keep the digestive system functioning at peak levels. Some women cannot tolerate grains in any form, gluten-free or not, so listen for signs of fatigue, excessive hunger, cravings, or digestive upset after you eat grains.

- Steer clear of alcohol, processed sugars, too much caffeine, and spicy foods, which can trigger hot flashes, aggravate urinary incontinence, increase mood swings, and trigger bone loss.

Intermittent Fasting in Menopause and Beyond

With cycling and perimenopause behind you, you can pursue intermittent fasting with few restrictions or time constraints. Many women practice it daily for weight loss, for weight maintenance, or for its health benefits. This is, oftentimes, the sweet spot for IF and women. You are no longer tethered to watching and waiting for a menstrual cycle each month, or worrying about supplies such as tampons or pads and schedules. You can much more easily integrate IF into your lifestyle.

For one thing, intermittent fasting helps slow down the aging process, because it regenerates your entire system starting with your cells and mitochondria, which I'm sure you'll be happy to hear. Moreover, intermittent fasting can help reduce hot flashes and many other uncomfortable symptoms.

There are lots of benefits of intermittent fasting for you at this stage in your life. A recap:

- More energy
- Weight loss and control and less hunger
- Increase in lean muscle mass, supported by proper diet and strength training
- Stronger immunity and less inflammation
- Protection against some diseases due to increased cell renewal
- Reduction in stress
- Improvement of insulin sensitivity in overweight women
- Less depression and anxiety
- Greater cognitive function

What's not to love? Women of all ages can benefit from intermittent fasting. However, it's important to learn how to practice intermittent fasting correctly and safely—which I cover in detail later in this book.

———————

Although each one of us experiences life in an individual way, I've observed that women who handle hormonal ups and downs the best are those who approach female changes as a natural progression of their lives rather than see them as a struggle. No matter what life stage you're in, now is the perfect time to look in the mirror and affirm to yourself, "I need to take care of myself now so I can have the quality of life I'm looking for."

To view the 19 references cited in this chapter,
please visit cynthiathurlow.com/references.

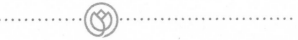

Part Two

The Intermittent Fasting Lifestyle

Chapter 6

. . . .

So—What Do I Eat?

Avoiding food for a certain time period is part of intermittent fasting—but so is eating food. When you practice intermittent fasting, you cluster your meals into a feeding window, typically an eight-hour time frame, but this can vary (see chapter 8). What you choose to eat in your feeding window takes on huge significance. You want to select the best, healthiest foods you can in order to support your hormones, feed your microbiome, maintain a healthy weight, encourage metabolic flexibility, and reduce inflammation.

When considering intermittent fasting, my patients and clients want to know above all: What can I eat? It's one of the most important questions, too, because all lifestyle changes start with proper food and nutrition. Your food choices are critical to your health and wellness and will help you be successful on my IF:45 plan and beyond.

So—back to the big question: What can you eat? The short answer is: *macros*. This term is short for macronutrients, and it refers to protein, carbohydrates, and fat, all of which should be part of a healthy, nutritious eating plan. (*Micro*nutrients, on the other hand, refer to vitamins and minerals.) To understand the whole picture, it's a good idea to break down, and understand, each macro.

Protein

Protein is foundational to good health. In fact, the name comes from the Greek word *proteos*, meaning "primary" or "first place."

This macro is commonly found in animal products, although it is present in other sources, such as nuts and legumes. It is made up of twenty compounds called amino acids, nine of which are essential, meaning that our bodies cannot make them. They must be obtained from food.

In the body, protein:

- Creates satiety so that you feel full after eating it
- Promotes growth and maintenance
- Stimulates biochemical reactions involving enzymes—proteins that regulate digestion, blood clotting, energy production, and muscle contraction
- Is a building block of hormones
- Forms the connective framework of many structures in the body
- Maintains the proper pH of the body (alkalinity and acidity)
- Regulates fluid balance
- Strengthens immune health
- Transports and stores nutrients
- Supplies energy

For the purpose of intermittent fasting, especially for women, the most important function of protein is building muscle mass. It's critical we take care of our muscles, because they are the largest site for glucose disposal, fatty acid oxidation, and cholesterol. As we get older, we tend to lose muscle (sarcopenia). To help prevent or slow the loss of muscle tissue, protein consumption is essential, so that the body can use amino acids to build muscle tissue, preserve the muscle we have, and help prevent sarcopenia.

A confusing point about protein is whether we get enough in our diets. The hard-and-fast truth is that most Americans, especially women, do not eat enough for an ideal body weight or for the needs of their muscle tissue. Unfortunately, most of the standard American diets are light on protein and heavy on seed oils and processed grains and sugars—and definitely not the way to support a healthy lifestyle or body composition.

Women need more protein. My clients are shocked when I tell them how much protein they should eat daily: the same amount of grams a day as your ideal body weight. If a healthy weight for your height and stature is 150 pounds, then your goal should be 150 grams of protein each day. Please do not get overwhelmed by this number. It might require some adjustments to your diet, but it is not impossible.

I prefer that you eat animal protein. It has the highest amino acid profile and best supports the growth and repair of muscles, hormones, enzymes, and antibodies. Red meat, in particular, has gotten a bad rap. But if you choose the grass-fed variety, it has a healthier omega-3 fatty acid profile and packages higher amounts of two key antioxidants, beta-carotene and vitamin E. What's more, grass-fed meat is higher in certain B vitamins such as riboflavin and thiamin.

Saturated Fat and Heart Disease

But what about the saturated fat in red meat and other foods? Does it elevate your chance of heart disease, particularly if you are at risk?

It's true that heart disease is the leading cause of death for women in the United States. What puts you at risk is having diabetes, being overweight or obese, eating an unhealthy diet, not exercising, drinking too much alcohol, or smoking.

As for eating saturated fat and heart disease, this is among the most controversial topics in all nutrition and the latest research is largely inconclusive. A 2015 review of this issue analyzed fifteen randomized controlled trials with over fifty-nine thousand participants. It found no statistically significant effects of reducing saturated fat in regard to heart attacks, strokes, or all-cause deaths. People who cut back on their saturated fat intake were just as likely to die, or suffer heart attacks or strokes, compared with those who ate more saturated fat.

The effect of saturated fat on the health of your heart also depends on the source of this fat. For example, a diet high in saturated fats in the form of fast food, fried products, sugary baked goods, and processed meats is likely to affect health differently than a diet high in saturated fats in the form of grass-fed meat and coconut.

My advice is always "moderation." Enjoy lean, grass-fed meats once or twice a week, if you wish, and talk to your doctor or cardiologist about this issue if you are at risk. The IF:45 plan will help you resolve issues that put you at risk, such as blood-sugar problems, weight concerns, and unhealthy eating patterns.

Aim for a variety of grass-fed, organic, pasture-raised animal protein. If you are concerned about cost, purchase foods you are able to afford and that fit your budget. Aldi's, Costco, and Trader Joe's often have organic animal protein at affordable prices. Sources of protein that are common in my house are beef, bison, chicken, shrimp, and eggs.

For my vegan and vegetarian friends, there are a variety of plant-based proteins available, including legumes, quinoa, nuts, and seeds. The quality of protein is different in plants than in animals, however. Yes, you can obtain the amino acids from plants but you'd have to eat a lot of plant food to obtain the same amount of protein in a piece of beef or chicken. For example, it takes 9 cups of cooked brown rice to equal the 40 grams of protein in a 5-ounce piece of lean beef! The caloric and carbohydrate load of the brown rice is huge—1,964 calories and 367 grams of carbs.

I've got to bring up soy. It constitutes a major protein source in plant-based diets. But please understand that soybean plants are largely genetically modified, and long-term exposure to GMOs can be detrimental to health.

Some examples of soy are tofu, edamame, and many vegan protein powders and bars. If you have a family history of estrogen-influenced cancers, like breast cancer, however, you may want to avoid soy. Soy can mimic estrogen in the body and possibly contribute to estrogen dominance. I generally suggest avoiding soy entirely, unless you choose fermented versions like natto or miso.

What about protein supplements? Be careful here, too. I found an article published by *Consumer Reports* sharing the findings of known toxins in various powders and drinks. Within the article and research performed by the Clean Label Project, "products made from sources of plant protein such as soy or hemp fared worse than those made from whey (milk) or egg, containing on average twice as much lead and measurably higher amounts of other contaminants."

The article went on to say: "Also important: Buying a product with an 'organic' label did not reduce the chances of getting a contaminated product. In fact, organic protein supplements had higher levels of heavy metals, on average, than nonorganic." Wow. These findings are definitely contrary to what the manufacturers would like us to believe.

Finally, when you start to eat any meal, I urge you to consume protein first, a healthy fat second, followed by vegetables and/or a carbohydrate. Eating in this order boosts satiety, helps balance your blood sugar and insulin, and feeds your brain.

Carbohydrates

Carbohydrate consumption is a hot topic. Should you eat carbs? Should you eat low-carb? What about no carbs?

Great questions. But first, what exactly is a "carb"? Carb is a shorthand expression for carbohydrate. Dietary carbohydrates fall into three main categories:

SUGARS. These are constructed of either single or double molecules of sugar and include glucose, fructose, galactose, and sucrose.

STARCHES. These are made of multiple numbers of sugar molecules, which eventually get broken down into glucose during digestion.

FIBER. Sometimes called roughage, fiber is the nondigestible portion of plants that can lower glucose and fat absorption, assist in weight control, and feed the healthy gut bacteria to promote a healthy microbiome.

Carbs are sometimes referred to as "simple" versus "complex," or "whole" versus "refined." Simple sugars are those found in table sugar, jams, candy, syrups, and processed foods, while "complex carbs" is simply another name for starches.

A more useful distinction is between whole carbs and refined carbs. Whole carbs are unprocessed and have not been refined in any way and contain the fiber found naturally in the food. Refined carbs have been processed, with the natural fiber and other nutrients removed or changed.

Examples of whole carbs include: non-starchy vegetables and starchy carbohydrates such as quinoa, legumes, winter squashes, potatoes, sweet potatoes, and whole grains. These carbs are high in nutrients, such as vitamins and minerals, required by the body to function optimally. They are also fiber-rich. Fiber keeps us full, plus helps escort harmful and excess estrogen from the body, for better hormonal balance.

Refined carbs are mostly the sugary foods I listed above, but also include white bread and any foods made with white flour. High in calories and low in nutrients, these foods lead to metabolic inflexibility, increase inflammation, trigger food cravings, alter our gut bacteria negatively, elevate blood sugar, and cause other problems.

Food quality is imperative, especially when you are intermittent fasting. You want to make sure that, in your feeding window, you are enjoying the most nutritious food possible, including carbohydrates.

Who Should Go Low-Carb?

There are little to no clear-cut definitions of what defines "low-carb." For example, if you are someone who normally eats the standard American diet (SAD), you might be consuming 300 grams a day of carbs. So if you reduced your carbs below that, your personal carb intake might be considered low-carb. "Low-carb" is quite bio-individual—and for that reason, I generally stay away from strict definitions of low-carb.

That said, here are three examples of what low-carb often looks like:

Ketogenic—under 30 grams a day

Low-carb—under 50 grams a day

Liberal—150 grams a day (if you're at this level, focus on eating
fewer carbs)

Under certain conditions, a low-carb eating plan complements inter-mittent fasting. I consider a low-carb diet to be one in which you eat 50 grams of carbs a day or less. Consider going low-carb if:

YOU HAVE A SIGNIFICANT AMOUNT OF WEIGHT TO LOSE. A low-carb plan helps your body burn its fat reserves for energy in preference to stored carbohydrates. The net result is weight loss. Just as intermittent fasting helps your body transition into a fat-burning mode, a low-carb diet pro-motes metabolic flexibility, helping your body switch over from burning carbs to burning fat.

YOU ARE INSULIN RESISTANT. A low-carb diet combined with intermit-tent fasting prompts your body to reduce insulin levels, preventing insulin resistance.

YOU ARE LEPTIN RESISTANT. When you overeat, your leptin levels are chronically high, and your brain doesn't recognize the "I'm full" signal. This is leptin resistance. It can be overcome with a low-carb diet, however. You lose weight, your leptin levels drop in response, and your cells are no longer resistant to leptin.

YOU MAY BE METABOLICALLY INFLEXIBLE. A low-carb diet encourages the body to burn fat as a fuel source and can help correct this condition.

A few cautions: For some women, low-carb diets followed over the long term can potentially impact thyroid function. Female hormones, es-pecially estrogen and progesterone, can either be instrumental in process-ing carbs efficiently or cause more fat to be stored. A bit of experimentation in terms of how many carbs you can eat daily is critical because we are all different.

Also, because it can be extremely restrictive, low-carb dieting is best done for a short period of time (no more than a few weeks)—or cyclically (on and off). This is where carb cycling comes in.

Carb Cycling

Carb cycling is an advanced dietary approach I use, in which you alternate higher carb intake with lower carb intake on a daily, weekly, or monthly basis. It has many benefits. Carb cycling:

- Regulates leptin and ghrelin for better appetite control
- Balances insulin more effectively and improves insulin sensitivity
- Promotes metabolic flexibility
- Assists in the conversion of the inactive thyroid hormone T4 to the active form T3, thus helping your metabolism
- Enhances fat-burning
- Helps you break weight-loss plateaus, in which weight loss has stalled
- Restocks muscle glycogen, which can be depleted by low-carb dieting and exercise
- Boosts your physical and athletic performance
- Provides flexibility in food selection and lets you enjoy carbs and leverage them for their benefits
- Creates variety and reminds the body that it is not starving (especially on higher-carb days).

With higher carbs, up to 50 percent of your daily intake would be quality carbs, especially on days when you're exercising with intensity or lifting weights. On my high-carb days, I consume more healthy carbs, and less fat, but I keep my protein intake about the same.

By contrast, a low-carb day would be a day when you aren't exercising as intensely or perhaps doing Pilates or yoga. Your carb intake would be around 25 percent of your daily caloric intake. The purpose of a low-carb cycle is to increase fat loss by lowering your insulin levels and help your body tap into fat stores for energy. On my low-carb days, I reduce my carbs and increase my healthy fats but keep my protein about the same.

Carb cycling is a part of the plan in the Optimization Phase, and a tool to use long-term for maintenance.

Use a Glucometer

I don't subscribe to a "one size fits all carb philosophy" as it pertains to intermittent fasting. Instead, I recommend using a device called a continuous glucose monitor (CGM) or a glucometer to check your glucose levels and how they respond to fasting, your diet, and your exercise program. I've been using the Nutrisense CGM monitor and app. It is easy and pain-free to apply. You can also use a blood glucometer, but these usually require finger pricking.

Whatever system you use, check your fasted morning level, which should optimally be 80–95 mg/dL or less. You can also test prior to eating and then thirty and sixty minutes afterward. In general, you want to maintain your glucose levels in the 80–90 mg/dL range. Important: If your blood sugar rises more than 30 points after a meal, it may be a sign that this meal had too many carbs. Dial back your carbs next time.

What you're trying to achieve is overall stability. If you are consistently seeing spikes up and over 100, especially after a meal, it may be a sign that you have consumed too many carbohydrates. Numbers above 100 are highly influenced by what you eat, stress, poor sleep, and illnesses, among other factors. If your number spikes to 140 after a meal, it may be a sign of insulin resistance, food intolerances, etc. Reduce the number of carbs and add more fat, like an extra avocado, or MCT oil.

CGM devices not only monitor your blood sugar but also your hunger cues. Here are some guidelines to help you do this:

Check your blood sugar when you feel hungry and track these feelings for three days. Record the readings and average them. The average is called your "trigger point." After the three-day tracking period, check your blood sugar to see if you are at your trigger point.

If you are at that point, eat; this means your gas tank is empty. If you are not, you still have energy to burn, and your gas tank is still full. Hold off breaking your fast or eating your next meal.

Because glucose is such a volatile fuel and effectively floats on top of all the fat in your body, measuring your blood sugar when you wake up or before you eat is an excellent way to ensure you are not chronically overfueling (from either fat or carbs).

Your pre-meal blood glucose trigger strongly correlates with your waking blood glucose. Rather than worrying about the rise in blood glucose after you eat, managing your blood glucose before you eat is much more useful if you want to lose fat and gain health!

Also, check your blood sugar after your meal. If it rises less than 30 points, your combination of protein/fat and carbs is good. If it rises over 30 points, you had too many carbs (quantity) and need to adjust next time. Or, avoid that particular carb and substitute a better choice such as a sweet potato, winter squash, beans, or legumes.

If your blood sugar regularly rises by more than 1.6 mmol/L (or 30 mg/dL) after meals, then it's likely you are eating excessive amounts of refined, processed carbohydrates and need to adjust your carbohydrate limit.

If you are cycling, an ideal time to consume more carbohydrates is during the luteal phase, especially the five to seven days prior to your menstrual cycle. At this time, you are more resistant to insulin, and you need to be strategic about the types of carbs you are consuming. This does not, however, mean excessive portions of carbs, just integration of an additional one or two servings daily that add up to 30 grams of quality carbs in a serving. Examples I often use are ⅓ cup of sweet potato or other root vegetable, ⅓ cup of winter squash, or ⅓ cup of beans or lentils.

All in all, carbohydrates are not the "bad guys" in nutrition, and they can definitely be included in your diet. For many people, it's difficult to stay on a low-carb or no-carb diet over the long term. It's better to learn how to enjoy carbs in a lasting, sustainable lifestyle that also meets your weight and body-mass goals. Please choose wisely and fully investigate what's best for your body.

Fats

Fats are classified according to their "saturation," a term that refers to the number of hydrogen atoms in their chains of fatty acids. When a fatty acid carries the maximum hydrogen atoms, it is said to be "saturated." The more saturated a fat, the more solid it is at room temperature. Examples of saturated fats include those found in beef, dairy products, butter, and some vegetables like coconuts.

If there are one or more places on the chain where hydrogens are missing, the fatty acid is unsaturated. A fatty acid with a single point of unsaturation is termed a monounsaturated fat. Examples are olive oil, olives, avocado, nuts, and seeds. A "polyunsaturated fat" is one with two or more points of unsaturation and includes many vegetable oils. The omega-3 fatty acids in fish are polyunsaturated fats.

Our bodies need fats for fuel and for the health of our organs, including the brain and the heart. Fats:

- Provide essential fatty acids—vitamin-like substances that have a protective effect on your body
- Help transport and distribute fat-soluble vitamins (A, D, E, and K)
- Form cellular membranes
- Insulate and protect your body
- Support growth and development
- Provide energy
- Regulate leptin so that it can tell your brain you're full
- Enhance the flavor of food

Fat and Hormone Balance

Fats are required for hormone production and regulation. While most hormones are secreted by glands, some are produced in fatty tissue as well. Estrogen is one example.

Cholesterol also plays a key role when it comes to our sex hormones. The body can't produce estrogen, progesterone, and testosterone without cholesterol. One of the ways your body manufactures cholesterol is from dietary fat. Yes, many people are afraid of high cholesterol, but low cholesterol can create many health issues, including cognitive impairment and hormonal imbalances. It all comes down to eating the right types of fat—which I call "healthy fat."

The healthiest types of fat you can enjoy for hormone balance are omega-3 fatty acids from fatty fish, flaxseeds, and chia seeds; avocado; coconut oil; olive oil; nuts; and nut butters. Organic, pasture-raised eggs are also an excellent source of healthy fat.

I do count saturated fats as healthy fats—those from lean, grass-fed courses and not from processed foods—because they support the production of sex hormones. It's true that eating saturated fat can increase unhealthy LDL cholesterol, but this elevation is usually accompanied by increases in good HDL cholesterol and decreases in triglycerides. A more serious culprit here is highly processed foods, such as sodas, white rice, white bread products, sugary cereals, sweets, and snack foods. They have been found to increase LDL cholesterol. As I noted in the sidebar on page 91, moderation is key. Some saturated fats, like those found in coconut oil, actually help your body burn fat.

Do not fixate on single macronutrients or micronutrients as the solution to a health problem or disease. Instead, take into consideration the nutrient quality of your entire diet. In other words, look at your diet holistically and concentrate on building healthful eating patterns.

That said, however, I emphasize that certain fats should be avoided, namely polyunsaturated fats found in some vegetable oils, also called seed oils. Found in many processed foods, they are high in omega-6 fatty acids, which increase free radicals and inflammation in the body. Among the offending fats in this category are seed oils such as soybean, peanut, corn, canola, cottonseed, sunflower, and safflower oils. I've learned that these oils can disrupt the health of your cellular membranes and mitochondria and keep them damaged for up to two years.

The Ideal Macro Ratio

Finding the right ratio of macros may take some time. It is different for everyone, especially if you still have your period and are changing your carb intake according to the phase of your cycle—or if you decide to carb cycle based on your activity level. But generally, I recommend a starting ratio of 50/30/20 (protein/fat/carbs) and adjusting as needed. How do you know if you have the right ratio for you? Ask yourself the following questions:

- How is your appetite? You should feel satiated after each meal and not feel like snacking. Nor should you have any sweet cravings.
- How is your energy level? It should feel stable and restored, not depleted, after each meal.
- How is your mental and emotional well-being? You should experience an improved well-being, a good mood, and mental energy after your meals. Your emotions should be positive, and your mind should be focused and clear.

Seriously consider these questions and listen to your body. Take, for example, my client Andrea. She had been navigating her forties pretty well until she started feeling sleepy after meals. Not long after that, her sleep was interrupted by night sweats. She was gaining weight around her abdomen, too.

Fluctuating hormones, as well as hormones surging at odd times during the month, were at the root of these changes, but so were her macro ratios. Andrea wasn't eating the right ratios to correct or support these hormonal transitions. She was eating too many poor-quality carbs, too little protein, and not enough healthy fat. I tweaked her diet by reducing her carbs while adding in a few healthy carbohydrates and increasing her protein and fat intake so that her daily ratio met the 50/30/20 level.

Then I started her on intermittent fasting—and voilà—Andrea regained her physical and mental energy after meals, lost the pesky pounds around her waistline, and began to feel like her old self again. Small nutritional tweaks made a big difference.

The meal plans in chapter 13 will help you with your macro ratios, plus they show you how to carb cycle. Follow these plans, and pretty soon, planning your own meals according to my recommendations will be second nature.

Got Hormone Imbalance? Seed Cycle!

I've mentioned seeds in this chapter, so I want to tell you about a fascinating and easy nutritional technique that works wonders for hormone balance: seed cycling. It is something you can do wherever you are in your hormonal journey. All it involves is eating different seeds throughout the month, and it makes a big impact on how you feel, especially if you have estrogen dominance. Here's what to do at each point in your cycle:

Days 1–14:

Eat flaxseeds and pumpkin seeds the first half of your cycle. Day 1 is the first day of your period. A tablespoon is all you need (daily) for this to work. These particular seeds help boost the production of estrogen.

Flaxseeds contain phytoestrogens, which are similar to estrogen, and pumpkin seeds are high in zinc, which has been known to help ease menstrual cramps.

Days 15–28:

Enjoy a combination of sunflower seeds and sesame seeds. Again, a tablespoon of each (daily) is all you need. These seeds help support the development of progesterone, which can help ease PMS symptoms. Simply add them to smoothies or salads, or make your own energy bites and granolas with these seeds. (Try my granola recipe on page 291.)

Both of these seeds are high in vitamin E, a nutrient that helps with hormone balance.

Expect to feel a noticeable improvement within two to three months of using this "seed cycling" strategy. This is such a fun way to feel better without the use of a prescription, and a good example of how wholesome food is medicine.

If you are no longer getting your period (not menstruating), you can still benefit from this strategy. Simply follow the lunar cycle. On the first day of a new moon, you would start on day 1 of the seed cycle.

Anti-inflammatory Nutrition and Hormone Balance

With the macros and foods I recommend on my meal plans, you'll be following an *anti-inflammatory* nutrition plan. This is extremely important for your health and for your hormones.

Inflammation, in and of itself, is not a bad thing. In fact, it's protective—the body's reaction to injury or illness. However, sometimes inflammation occurs chronically and can cause problems such as hormone imbalances and poor regulation of hormones.

Inflammation is also the root cause of most chronic illnesses, including heart disease, cancer, Alzheimer's, thyroid disorders, digestive diseases like Crohn's, and IBS. Not to mention, autoimmune diseases like Hashimoto's thyroiditis, rheumatoid arthritis, and fibromyalgia!

Diet is very much responsible for most of the inflammation in your body. So the first step to staying healthy and protecting your body is anti-inflammatory nutrition.

Before I get into specific foods that help decrease inflammation, here's a list of foods that are scientifically proven to create inflammation and should be avoided:

GLUTEN. A protein found in wheat, barley, and rye, gluten can mount an immune attack against the body's own cells, otherwise known as autoimmunity. This can cause "small intestine hyperpermeability," otherwise known as leaky gut, in which gaps in the intestinal walls allow bacteria and other toxins to pass into the bloodstream, triggering a further autoimmune cascade in other areas of the body.

Implicated in thyroid disorders, gluten can aggravate Hashimoto's disease by inflaming the thyroid gland. The problem is known as "molecular mimicry." It basically means that your body's immune system is attacking not only the gluten but also its own tissue.

REFINED SUGAR. This refers to sugar that has been stripped from plant sources and therefore devoid of the context of the plant nutrients. Table sugar and high-fructose corn syrup (in soft drinks and other processed foods) are two notable examples, but there are others added to food (see the sidebar below).

These sugars raise blood glucose levels, which in turn spike an insulin response, and can be stored as fat if your body has exceeded storage sites for excessive sugar in your liver and skeletal muscles.

There are many health risks related to eating too much sugar: heart disease, diabetes, and cancer; depression; aging both in cells and in your skin; metabolic inflexibility; and weight gain.

And of course, the more sugar you take in, the more of it you must process, and that requires more insulin—possibly leading to insulin resistance. Problems with insulin resistance and blood-sugar regulation can cause imbalances of the key reproductive hormones, including estrogen, testosterone, LH, and FSH.

A significant part of the reason for such widespread health damage has to do with inflammation. Sugar is highly inflammatory.

A 2018 review published in the journal *Nutrients* linked the consumption of more dietary sugar—especially from sugary drinks—with chronic inflammation. People with higher sugar diets had more inflammatory markers in their blood, including a marker called C-reactive protein.

Sneaky Names for Sugar on Food Labels

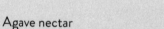

- Agave nectar
- Barbados sugar (also called muscovado sugar)
- Barley malt & barley malt syrup
- Beet sugar
- Brown sugar
- Cane juice & cane juice crystals (sometimes called dehydrated or evaporated cane juice)
- Cane sugar
- Caramel
- Carob syrup

- Coconut sugar (or coconut/palm sugar)
- Confectioners' sugar (or powdered/icing sugar)
- Corn sweetener/syrup & corn syrup solids
- D-ribose
- Date sugar
- Demerara sugar
- Dextrin
- Dextrose
- Fructose & crystalline fructose
- Fruit juice & fruit juice concentrate
- Galactose
- Glucose & glucose solids
- Granulated sugar
- Grape sugar
- High-fructose corn syrup (HFCS)
- Honey
- Hydrolyzed starch
- Invert sugar (or liquid invert sugar)
- Malt syrup
- Maltodextrin
- Maltol
- Maltose
- Mannose
- Maple syrup
- Molasses
- Raw sugar
- Refiners' sirup
- Rice syrup (or brown rice syrup)
- Saccharose
- Sorghum syrup
- Sucrose ("table sugar")
- Sweet potato syrup

- Sweet sorghum
- Tapioca syrup
- Treacle
- Turbinado sugar

DAIRY. The purpose of milk is to make calves gain weight quickly. And because we are not baby cows—or even babies anymore—our bodies don't require milk. Contrary to popular belief and ads, you don't necessarily build bone strength from the calcium in milk and other dairy products; you can get calcium from a lot of plant foods. In fact, cow dairy is a highly inflammatory food for most people. The processing it goes through, especially to make skim milk, does not make it more nutritious, only more inflammatory. Plus, many dairy foods contain a protein called the A1 casein protein, now thought to create a range of digestive and health issues.

SEED OILS. On average, Americans get 80 percent of their fat calories from seed oils. These include canola, corn, cottonseed, grapeseed, rice bran, safflower, soybean, and sunflower oils. Soybean oil, in particular, is the most consumed oil in the United States. All of these oils are high in unstable omega-6 fatty acids that break down into toxins when you cook with them.

In ancient times, humans obtained omega-3 and omega-6 fatty acids in a certain ratio that has been estimated to have been about 1:1. However, in the past century or so, this ratio has shifted dramatically due to the Western diet and may be as high as 20:1 (omega-6 fatty acids to omega-3 fatty acids). Too many omega-6 fatty acids relative to omega-3s contributes to chronic inflammation, which damages the lining of blood vessels, affecting overall circulation, blood flow to the brain, and risks for heart disease and diabetes. The fatty acids in seed oils also generate a tremendous amount of free radicals—chaotic molecules that damage cells

There are other problems with seed oils. With excessive consumption, they disrupt metabolism and create metabolic disorders such as type 2 diabetes. At a certain concentration, these fatty acids shut down the ability of the mitochondria to generate energy. To survive, they're forced to draw more sugar from the bloodstream, which greatly depletes your blood sugar. When your blood sugar drops, you get hypoglycemia (low blood sugar) and powerful sugar cravings. So a diet high in seed oils can actually get you hooked on sugar and processed carbohydrates!

The easiest way to avoid these problems is to not consume seed oils. Also, read labels, because seed oils show up in many processed foods. Stick to the healthy fats I talk about throughout this book, and you'll go a long way toward preventing the health issues caused by seed oils.

CHEMICAL FOOD ADDITIVES. Most processed foods are laced with chemicals—"additives"—designed to preserve shelf life, add color or artificial flavor, thicken the food, manipulate the taste, or otherwise tinker with the food in some way. Many of these additives alter microbes in the gut, creating an environment favorable for serious illnesses. Our bodies have built-in defenses against harmful bacteria, but chemically created food additives slip past these safeguards. Normally, the mucus lining of the gut protects the intestines from an influx of bad bacteria, but additives stealthily transport harmful bacteria across the intestinal lining, negatively altering the gut environment. If these changes are severe, inflammation can set in. It can create leaky gut, irritable bowel disorder (IBD), and even colorectal cancer.

So naturally you'll want to shun foods that have inflammation-producing properties, since they can cause widespread damage to the body.

Select Anti-inflammatory Foods

Fortunately, there are more anti-inflammatory foods from which to choose than those that create inflammation.

Fruits and Vegetables

It's hard to say enough about the anti-inflammatory powers of this wide-ranging group of foods. Any one you eat is bound to make an impact on preventing inflammation, although, based on research, we want to strive for brightly pigmented options. Some with known potential include dark leafy greens such as spinach, kale, and collard greens—all of which are low-carb and contain a variety of vitamins and minerals that protect against cellular damage. Green veggies also contain natural plant compounds called isoflavonoids that help your liver quickly excrete harmful, excess estrogen. Furthermore, all of the cruciferous vegetables have potent antioxidant activity for fighting inflammation. Berries are the superstars of the fruit world due to their high concentration of antioxidants, especially vitamin C, an overall inflammation fighter. Berries also can help your body produce more serotonin.

Whole Grains

Certain whole grains are considered anti-inflammatory because they actually reduce the levels of C-reactive protein in the blood (a marker for inflammation). It's best to choose gluten-free varieties such as brown rice, quinoa, amaranth, buckwheat, millet, teff, sorghum, and certified gluten-free oats, but eat them in small quantities, especially if you are over age forty. With age, the body does not process grains well.

Personally, I eat grain-free as much as possible. Grains and my digestive system do not go together well. I believe this has a lot to do with the generations of genetically modified grains that we have available in the US market. Most of my carbohydrate intake comes from vegetables and fruits.

Healthy Fats

Please don't be scared of all fat. Fat fear is an old dogma that needs to be eradicated. Healthy fats are essential to proper cellular function and vitamin absorption. They can be found in nuts and seeds, especially walnuts, which are chock-full of omega-3s and nutrients like manganese, copper, and magnesium that help repair damage done by inflammation.

Olive oil is a fantastic healthy fat, and lots of research shows that people who eat olive oil regularly have less cancer and heart disease. Harvard scientists found that women in Greece who ate olive oil more than once a day had 25 percent lower breast cancer rates than women eating the oil less frequently. The healing power of olive oil is believed to come from its monounsaturated fat content. It helps reduce inflammation. You want to purchase organic, cold-pressed extra-virgin olive oil for best results.

Avocados guard against inflammation, too. Much of the fat in avocados is monounsaturated, too, and thus health-protective. This food is very high in glutathione, the "master antioxidant" with formidable power to destroy free radicals. It also stops toxins from doing harm.

Coconut oil is a great choice, too. Substituting 2 tablespoons of this oil for other fats you might normally eat can help you pare 60 percent more abdominal fat every month, reported the *American Journal of Clinical Nutrition*.

Many types of coconut oil contain medium-chain triglycerides, a type of fatty acid that stimulates your liver to burn stored abdominal fat for energy. The best form of MCT oil is one containing "C-8," a fatty acid that burns fat, boosts energy, enhances brain function, improves the microbiome, regulates appetites, and supports metabolism.

Another fatty acid in coconut oil—lauric acid—has anti-inflammatory properties.

Fatty Fish and Seafood

Eat omega-3-rich wild Alaskan salmon, sardines, tuna, and mackerel several times a week for their heart-healthy, anti-inflammatory benefits. Including about 12 ounces of seafood in your weekly diet can help reduce stiffness and aches (caused by inflammation) in your joints and tendons by as much as 55 percent, research shows. These fats are not to be confused with omega-6 fatty acids, as I described above. The ratio of omega-6 fats to omega-3 fats in the diet should be 1:1, if looking at traditional hunter-gatherers. Most Americans consume far too many omega-6 fats and not enough omega-3 fats. The standard American diet ratio is 20:1 (omega-6/omega-3). Include more omega-3 fats into your diet and it will help keep the omega-6 fats in better balance.

Cooked Asian Mushrooms

Asian mushrooms, especially shiitake mushrooms, contain substances that boost immunity and discourage inflammation. A 2018 review of the anti-inflammatory properties of edible mushrooms concluded: "Recent reports indicate that edible mushroom extracts exhibit favorable therapeutic and health-promoting benefits, particularly in relation to diseases associated with inflammation. In all certainty, edible mushrooms can be referred to as a 'superfood' and are recommended as a valuable constituent of the daily diet."

Herbs and Spices

Turmeric, in particular, is known for its anti-inflammatory properties. This deep orange spice is popular in Indian and Southeast Asian cooking and contains a powerful compound called curcumin, the anti-inflammatory effect of which is said to rival that of Motrin and other anti-inflammatory drugs. Garlic, ginger, and cinnamon are other power players in this category. They block the formation of harmful inflammation inside your arteries.

Individualize Your Choices

In any healthy eating plan, including one designed to address inflammation, aim for variety. Include as many whole foods as possible and always eat an abundance of fruits and veggies.

Not all of these foods may agree with you. I'm a good example, and I've had firsthand experience with this issue. After a trip to Hawaii with my husband in 2019, I came back home writhing with the worst abdominal pain of my life. I suffered a ruptured appendix, inflammation throughout my colon, a small bowel obstruction, abscesses in my peritoneum (abdominal cavity), and a fistula (an abnormal tunnel between my appendix and cecum). I was a mess. I had to wait six weeks to have surgery to remove my appendix because I had been so life threateningly ill.

After I got out of the hospital, the doctor recommended a "low residue" diet. Typically, this diet means eating highly processed foods, the type of foods I truly don't eat and don't recommend to my clients. The only healthy foods included in this suggested way of eating were well-cooked meats (think stewed and roasted meat) and boiled vegetables. So that's what I focused on. Eating this way gave my digestive system time to heal and allowed me to consume nutrient-dense foods without much difficulty. I did miss other foods but slowly adapted. I embraced a carnivore-type lifestyle (mostly meats) for the first nine months out of the hospital but was grateful to start slowly increasing other foods over the next year.

What I discovered was that my gut was very sensitive to foods I had previously loved eating—nuts, seeds, and fruits. I also found that I was highly sensitive to green leafy vegetables, so I had to eliminate those. These foods, along with nuts, contain oxalates, which can bind to minerals in the gut and prevent the body from absorbing them. High-oxalate foods may also increase the risk of kidney stones in susceptible people. But not everyone has a problem with oxalates.

Going forward, I was able to stick to my pre-surgery practice of avoiding gluten, grains, and dairy. And I could still eat eggs, beef, pork, bison, fish, and poultry. All of these strategies worked for me, and this is how I eat from day to day. After one year, I managed to regain most of the weight I lost during my thirteen-day hospitalization. I'm sleeping well, too, and have great energy. My point is that you may have to tweak some of these recommendations for your own unique bio-individuality.

Although all of the foods listed above are technically anti-inflammatory, if you have a leaky gut or other issues and haven't been tested for food sensitivity, you might be experiencing inflammation even from something as sublime as an avocado. I urge you to do your own personal research, keep a food diary, and try an elimination diet if you have symptoms of chronic inflammation that don't seem to be subsiding.

I believe in substantial testing and use the mediator release test (MRT) blood test on my clients to determine food sensitivities. It checks your immune system response (or non-response) to 150 foods and chemicals. I also use the GI-MAP (DNA-based stool testing) and DUTCH (dried urine and saliva testing for hormones).

The important point about diet is also to obtain the proper macronutrients—proteins, fats, and carbohydrates—timed around your fasting and feeding windows. You'll learn how to do that when we get to my IF:45 plan in part 3.

To view the 17 references cited in this chapter,
please visit cynthiathurlow.com/references.

Chapter 7

. . . .

How to Supplement While Fasting

While intermittent fasting, you're giving your body a break from food—and all the benefits that go with it—burning fat, balancing your hormones, countering aging, and more big benefits.

But what about supplements? Can you take them while fasting and following the IF:45 plan? The answer is yes, but you have to understand:

Which supplements can be taken on empty stomach
Which supplements should be taken with food
What supplements will provoke an insulin spike
What substances can break your fast
How hydration fits into intermittent fasting

Understanding each one of these issues is essential for getting the best results and tapping into the intrinsic benefits of intermittent fasting.

Take my patient Sally, for example. She had been using intermittent fasting as a strategy for about six months but was not seeing results. It wasn't until we took a careful look at her fasting habits that we found out why.

For one thing, Sally was drinking fatty, sugary coffees daily during her fasting window. She was "sneaking" gum, candy, and even certain supplements into her fasted periods—all of which tricked her system into believing that food was coming. Consequently, her body wasn't burning fat. And during her feeding window, she confessed to snacking between meals.

Once she understood how these things were adversely impacting her results, she changed her habits and her success with intermittent fasting skyrocketed! Her brain fog disappeared, she had more energy, and she was able to fit back into her "skinny" jeans again. Small, subtle tweaks made a huge difference.

Supplements taken correctly on the IF:45 plan can actually improve your results. So let's talk about what supplements to include and when, hydration, and a little bit about the science behind fasting and supplementing.

Water—Drink Up! (with Electrolytes)

Staying hydrated while fasting (and while feeding) is absolutely critical. Every cell in your body needs water, and every metabolic process uses it. You must consistently hydrate, because there is no backup storage in the body for water like there is for food.

Also, during the Induction Phase of my IF:45 plan, you'll be reducing your carbohydrate intake. Because of diuresis, this releases a lot of water from your cells—water that needs to be replaced. Staying hydrated also helps curb any possible hunger, improves mental clarity, and promotes gut health.

Also, our thirst sensation declines with age, increasing the risk of dehydration. With dehydration comes the loss of elasticity in your skin (which contributes to wrinkles and sagging)—so drink up whether you feel thirsty or not.

Aim for up to half your body weight in ounces of water daily, supplemented with electrolytes (see page 119), which, among other functions, help keep you hydrated.

So—always hydrate, fasting or not!

Enjoy Other Beneficial Fluids

You may also drink coffee and herbal teas. If you like coffee, it is a very beneficial beverage to include while fasting, especially in the morning. It induces autophagy and benefits cellular metabolism. It can also boost your metabolism, enhance fat-burning, and protect your brain cells.

What's more, coffee is an appetite suppressant. It contains plant antioxidants called chlorogenic acids that can help reduce hunger. The caffeine in coffee will do the same because of the metabolism boost it provides. Coffee also contains PYY (peptide tyrosine tyrosine), a hormone that can suppress hunger. It is released into blood cells in the lining of the small intestine and colon and, in essence, helps you feel full and satiated.

But what if you're sensitive to caffeine? You can curb your hunger and suppress your appetite with decaf coffee, too. In fact, for taming your appetite, one study found that decaffeinated coffee was more effective for suppressing appetite than caffeinated because it caused a sharper rise in PYY.

Be careful about drinking too much coffee, though. Some people, because of bio-individuality, are sensitive to it. Excess coffee can raise both cortisol and blood sugar, for example. Additionally, you also might take in mycotoxins—toxins produced by fungus and found in most commercial coffee and other foods, particularly grains. Fortunately, mycotoxins are neutralized by your liver as long as your exposure remains low. And although their levels are far below safety limits and too low to be of practical significance, overdosing on coffee could be a problem. Excessive mycotoxin exposure can be harmful to the brain and kidneys by causing inflammation and suppressing the immune system.

As for green or black teas, they also stimulate autophagy, especially in the liver, due to their EGCG (epigallocatechin-3-gallate) content. A potent polyphenol, EGCG is thought to reduce inflammation, help with weight loss, and play a role in preventing heart and brain disease.

Tea in general is also a potential longevity agent, mostly because it is very high in antioxidants that defuse free radical attacks, thwarting aging. In a study conducted by the National Institute of Nutrition in Rome, participants drank slightly more than a cup of strong tea brewed for two minutes with three teaspoons of either black or green tea leaves. Tests revealed that antioxidant activity in the tea drinkers' blood soared by 41 to 48 percent within just thirty minutes after they drank the green tea and fifty minutes after the black tea.

The antioxidant power of tea has been well documented in many other research studies, especially when it comes to cardiovascular disease. Experiments show that tea blocks the buildup of plaque, reduces the risk of stroke, and prevents abnormal blood clotting.

Drinking either green or black tea may even halt the spread of cancer. Rutgers researchers discovered that natural chemicals in tea blocked the ability of leukemia and liver tumor cells to make DNA, necessary to reproduce themselves. Thus, the cancer cells could not proliferate and spread tumors.

Green tea, specifically, has a great reputation as a fat burner—for good reason. The EGCG in tea can enhance metabolism, for one thing. Also, animal studies suggest that EGCG can boost the effects of some fat-burning hormones, such as norepinephrine. EGCG blocks an enzyme that breaks down norepinephrine. When this enzyme is inhibited, more norepinephrine is secreted and thus promotes the breakdown of fat. In fact, caffeine and EGCG—both of which are found naturally in green tea—may have a synergistic fat-burning effect. Your fat cells can break down more fat, which is released into your bloodstream to be burned off for energy.

So yes—enjoy all the tea you want on the IF:45 plan!

Other good teas to choose include bergamot tea, unsweetened herbal teas, and ginger tea. They, too, have polyphenols and other compounds that stimulate autophagy. As with coffee, these teas can help stimulate metabolism and weight loss. Enjoy them as part of your intermittent fast, and make sure to purchase organic varieties to help avoid toxin exposure.

But enjoy them plain—no milk, cream, creamers, sugar, or even artificial sweeteners—while fasting. During your feeding window, it is fine to have a little milk, cream, or sugar—if that is how you prefer your beverage and can tolerate dairy. But generally, it is a good idea to avoid these, especially sugar and artificial sweeteners.

Clean Fasts versus Dirty Fasts

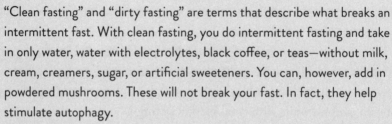

"Clean fasting" and "dirty fasting" are terms that describe what breaks an intermittent fast. With clean fasting, you do intermittent fasting and take in only water, water with electrolytes, black coffee, or teas—without milk, cream, creamers, sugar, or artificial sweeteners. You can, however, add in powdered mushrooms. These will not break your fast. In fact, they help stimulate autophagy.

Generally, dirty fasting is when you consume food or beverages, like cream, butter, non-nutrient sweeteners, or low-calorie foods during your fasting window and assume they are benign. It is generally accepted that consuming food during your fasting window will break a clean fast and potentially evoke an insulin response and disrupt autophagy.

Remember Sally above? She had been dirty fasting, and it completely stalled her progress.

The Problem with Artificial Sweeteners

You'd think that artificial sweeteners like stevia, sucralose, aspartame, and others would be okay on a fast because they contain no calories. But no—they are not okay, especially while fasting.

Artificial sweeteners are synthetic chemicals that stimulate sweet taste receptors on the tongue. Stevia comes from the stevia plant, which is not artificial. However, you need to be careful. Lots of companies add in other sweeteners, such as sucrose and sugar alcohols to their stevia products.

Artificial sweeteners are found everywhere, from diet soft drinks and desserts to packaged meals and low-calorie desserts. They are even found in non-food items, such as chewing gum and toothpaste.

The big question with artificial sweeteners is: Will they provoke an insulin response and therefore break your fast?

Sometimes insulin is released even before any sugar or carbs enter your bloodstream. This response is known as "cephalic phase insulin release." It is triggered by the sight, smell, and taste of food, as well as chewing and swallowing. So when you hear someone say, "I gain weight by just looking at food," there is some truth behind this statement!

Remember that if blood-sugar levels drop too low, our livers release stored glycogen to stabilize it. This happens when we fast, even overnight. There are a couple of theories on how artificial sweeteners may interfere with this process:

1. The sweet taste of artificial sweeteners triggers the cephalic phase insulin release, causing a small rise in insulin levels.
2. Using artificial sweeteners on a regular basis negatively alters the balance of good gut bacteria to bad bacteria. This may create insulin resistance, leading to both increased blood sugar and higher insulin levels.

Only a few studies have been conducted on artificial sweeteners and insulin response. Based on what is known, probably the biggest offender is sucralose. In one study, seventeen people were given either sucralose or water. Afterward, they underwent a glucose tolerance test. Those given sucralose had 20 percent higher blood insulin levels. They also cleared the insulin from their bodies more slowly. It is believed that sucralose increases insulin levels by triggering receptors in the mouth—the cephalic phase insulin release.

Saccharin may do the same, although there are few high-quality human trials on this sweetener. Acesulfame-K raises insulin in rats, but to date, no human studies have been conducted on this effect. Aspartame produces no effect on insulin but has many other adverse effects on the body, such as headaches, dizziness, unexplainable mood swings, vomiting and nausea, and abdominal cramps.

As for stevia, it does not contain anything that could cause an insulin response, and, technically speaking, it does not break a fast. This doesn't mean you should use it, however. All sweeteners, including stevia, are known to trigger hunger and make you crave sugar—two factors we are trying to eliminate with intermittent fasting. Their sweet taste fools your body into thinking it will get some sugary, high-calorie foods—but it's not getting any. This drives your appetite, instigates cravings, and makes it harder to satisfy your hunger.

So if you're looking to control hunger, cure your sugar addiction, and lose weight, one of the most effective strategies is to cut out artificial sweetness altogether.

Who Shouldn't Practice Intermittent Fasting?

Many people try intermittent fasting to lose weight, and others use the method to address chronic conditions such as hormonal issues, gut problems, mental clarity, or joint problems. But intermittent fasting isn't for everyone. Some people should steer clear of it:

- Children and teens under age eighteen
- The elderly
- Women who are pregnant or breastfeeding or trying to conceive
- People with a severe form of diabetes called brittle diabetes OR any diabetic who is unaware of when their blood sugar is low (hypoglycemia)
- Those being treated for serious liver, kidney, cardiovascular, or lung issues
- Those with a history of eating disorders (anorexia, bulimia, binge eating, or a combination of these)
- People with a low body weight, generally diagnosed as a body mass index of below 18.5. BMI is calculated from our height and weight to give us a general measure of our body fat. The Centers for Disease Control and Prevention (CDC) considers a score below 18.5 as underweight.

- Female athletes in training for a competition
- Anyone who has been recently hospitalized
- Anyone who is struggling with alcoholism
- Anyone undergoing significant or prolonged stress, which should be resolved prior to fasting

Electrolytes

A group of substances you are flushing out of your body when you fast, along with water, is electrolytes. These are minerals such as sodium, potassium, magnesium, and chloride. Affecting every cell in your body, they carry electrical impulses that allow your cells to communicate and perform basic functions. They all work together, too. If you do not get enough sodium, for example, you cannot absorb magnesium. So balancing electrolytes is essential!

When you start fasting, you might experience side effects like headaches, nausea, body aches, insomnia, and a collection of symptoms commonly referred to as "keto flu." These are usually related to a mild electrolyte imbalance and can be corrected by supplementing with electrolytes. Here is a closer look at these important minerals.

Sodium and Potassium

One of the most important electrolytes is sodium. In a fasted state or while on a low-carb diet, you can lose sodium in your urine. This is initiated by the renin-angiotensin-aldosterone system (RAAS), a hormone system that regulates blood pressure and fluid balance.

RAAC is mainly comprised of the three hormones renin, angiotensin II, and aldosterone. Renin is a hormone produced in the kidneys. It raises blood pressure and retains sodium. Angiotensin II is a protein that increases blood pressure, body water, and sodium content.

Aldosterone is responsible for keeping the sodium-potassium-water balance in the blood. This hormone works by mainly preserving sodium content. When the body thinks it needs more sodium, it releases aldosterone and puts the body into "sodium conservation" mode. This forces your body to retain more sodium and reduces the amount of sodium you lose in your sweat.

When you have too much aldosterone, you can end up with excess sodium and lower levels of potassium. The excess ends up in the bloodstream, forcing your heart to pump harder, which can then result in high blood pressure. Recent studies have pointed out that those who overproduce aldosterone also have insulin resistance.

Low aldosterone levels can be linked to low sodium levels, and the salt craving we get is a sign that our body needs sodium. So in a way, aldosterone acts as a messenger, telling your kidneys to keep enough salt for the body's internal processes.

When you fast, you not only lose water, but you also deplete sodium. If you lose too much sodium, a number of things can happen. Low sodium can increase cortisol and epinephrine, causing insomnia and other stress responses. Other symptoms of low sodium include:

- Weakness
- Headaches
- Nausea
- Restlessness
- Insulin resistance

Magnesium

Magnesium participates in more than three hundred reactions in the body. But chances are, you don't get enough magnesium in your diet, even though this mineral is widely distributed in nuts, seeds, legumes, and other foods. One study found that ten out of eleven apparently healthy women were magnesium-deficient based on a special oral magnesium test. The authors concluded: "The results showed there are more frequent deficiencies of magnesium in organisms than it is generally assumed."

Deficiencies are generally caused by chronic diseases, medications such as antibiotics and diabetes drugs, processed foods, excessive alcohol usage, stress, and magnesium-depleted soils (even if organically farmed). Another reason we are not getting enough of it is because of our water supply. Our ancient ancestors used to obtain magnesium from their water, but our water supply is completely devoid of magnesium. Plus, a lot of people now drink bottled water, which has zero magnesium.

An ongoing shortfall of magnesium can cause muscle spasms and pain, insomnia, and fatigue. More serious consequences include high blood pressure; calcifications in the heart, liver, and skeletal muscles; kidney disease; and heart disease.

As for intermittent fasting, why is magnesium important?

For one thing, the mitochondria can be damaged in the absence of adequate magnesium. We do not want to disrupt these cellular factories, or else we disrupt their ability to create energy, and we open the door to mitochondrial disorders.

Also, a shortfall of magnesium can make you more vulnerable to insulin resistance—a condition we are trying to prevent and correct with fasting. In a statistical study of thirteen clinical trials published in 2017 in *Nutrients*, supplementation with magnesium reduced insulin resistance in insulin-resistant patients who were deficient in this important mineral. Many medical experts believe that magnesium may help intervene in the course of diabetes, which is preceded by untreated insulin resistance.

Magnesium is also being looked at as a natural way to curb food cravings. It has been discovered in research that if you are deficient in this mineral, you may experience more food cravings. A suggested dosage of 600 milligrams of magnesium daily has been shown to significantly reduce food cravings.

Magnesium is also important for bone strength—a concern for women going through perimenopause and menopause. Women prone to osteoporosis often lack adequate magnesium. It works with calcium and vitamin D to keep bones from deteriorating.

Magnesium in general has a huge impact on other areas of your health. A 2015 review published in *Nutrients* noted that low levels of magnesium have been associated with a number of chronic diseases, such as Alzheimer's disease, type 2 diabetes, high blood pressure, cardiovascular disease, migraines, and attention deficit hyperactivity disorder (ADHD).

There are ten types of magnesium supplements that target different tissues. The most absorbable—and therefore the best used and digested by the body—are listed in the chart below. I generally recommend both oral and transdermal (through the skin) magnesium products for the best absorption. I suggest using transdermal magnesium two or three times a week; oral formulations can be taken daily and the dosage is largely based on needs. For example, can you tolerate the dosage recommended by the manufacturer? Or are you constipated and need a higher dose? These are issues to discuss with your health care practitioner.

The Most Bioavailable Forms of Magnesium and How to Use Them

FORMS OF MAGNESIUM	USES AND BENEFITS
Magnesium chloride	• Treats constipation • Soothes heartburn
Magnesium citrate	• Treats constipation • Supports energy production in the body
Magnesium glycinate	• Acts as an anti-inflammatory agent • Treats constipation • May help reduce anxiety, depression, stress, and insomnia
Magnesium lactate	• Is gentler on the digestive system than other forms of magnesium
Magnesium malate	• Is gentler on the digestive system than other forms of magnesium • May help resolve chronic fatigue
Magnesium orotate	• May promote heart health
Magnesium L-threonate	• May help manage certain brain disorders, such as depression and age-related memory loss

Chloride

This member of the electrolyte family is not a mineral you read much about, but it is important to your health nonetheless. It works in partnership with sodium and potassium to help control fluids within the body and maintain electrolyte balance. Like sodium, chloride influences muscle function and helps maintain proper blood pressure.

Chloride is usually paired with sodium in ordinary table salt, otherwise known as sodium chloride. Because it is in most foods, chloride deficiencies are rare. In the form of hydrochloric acid, chloride makes up part of gastric juice in the stomach and helps the body digest and absorb essential nutrients from food.

Supplementing with Electrolytes

Because of this intricate interplay of the RAAS and electrolytes, it is critical to supplement with these minerals. Well-balanced electrolytes will help you achieve a better fasting state and help you maintain a successful fast.

I recommend electrolyte products that dissolve in water, and I have mine first thing in the morning. Make sure that you use unflavored electrolytes that can be dissolved in water while fasting. A flavored product will break your fast.

And, during your feeding window, salt your foods. Yes, you heard me right! We also need salt in our diets to help maintain our electrolyte balance.

Other Supplements for Successful Fasting

According to the latest scientific evidence, there are several specific supplements that you can take while fasting that will enhance your fasting experience. Some are actual food products that will not break your fast but rather will support it. Although I recommend supplements and they promote successful fasting, they are entirely optional.

Spermidine

Spermidine is a supplement that protects your brain and your heart and mimics the same effects on human cells as fasting. Originally discovered in semen, which gives this supplement its name, it is a polyamine—a chemical compound with molecules composed of at least two amino groups. There are more than two hundred research articles in the National

Library of Medicine (PubMed) that report on the health and longevity benefits of spermidine. Specifically, spermidine:

- Improves the oxidative pathway for energy
- Helps autophagy
- Reduces methionine, which in high levels can alter DNA
- Fights free radicals, which can damage cells and create oxidative stress
- Increases mitochondria in the heart
- Increases macrophages, a type of white blood cell of the immune system that engulfs and digests cellular debris, germs, cancer cells, and other harmful foreign substances
- Reduces inflammatory cytokines, molecules that promote inflammation
- Increases stem cell activity to assist the body's regenerative processes
- Affords more cellular protection
- Reduces white fatty tissue
- Reduces sarcopenia
- Protects against cardiovascular disease and cancer when levels are increased

For all these wonderful benefits to kick in, your microbiome needs to be healthy with a good population of friendly gut bacteria, and your digestion should be operating well. Also, levels in the body decrease as we age.

Spermidine is found naturally in various foods: natto, miso, beef, mushrooms, salmon, roe, and chicken.

I recommend and use a product called Spermidine Life by Longevity Labs. The dosage is two capsules daily.

Berberine

Tested in hundreds of different studies, berberine helps lower blood sugar, stimulate weight loss, and improve heart health, to name a few benefits. It is one of the few supplements shown to be as effective as a pharmaceutical drug, namely metformin (Glucophage), prescribed to reduce blood sugar in people with type 2 diabetes.

Berberine is a compound found primarily in the barberry plant, and it offers many medicinal benefits. Berberine:

- Decreases insulin resistance, making insulin more effective
- Helps the body break down sugars inside cells
- Decreases sugar production in the liver
- Slows the breakdown of carbohydrates in the gut
- Increases the number of beneficial bacteria in the gut.
- Helps the body get into autophagy sooner
- May be effective as a weight-loss supplement.

It is common to take 500 milligrams, three times per day (a total of 1,500 milligrams per day). Although this supplement has many benefits, be sure to discuss it with a member of your health care team prior to starting it, especially if you take prescription medications on a daily basis or have a history of diabetes or hypoglycemia.

Chromium GTF

Chromium GTF is technically referred to as chromium polynicotinate. It is chromium that is chemically bound to natural vitamin B3 (niacin).

This is a simple, inexpensive mineral supplement that can work for weight loss, lower your appetite, reduce body fat, increase lean body mass, boost immune functioning, and help get your blood sugar under control.

I occasionally recommend chromium GTF because it induces many desirable bodily changes that align with intermittent fasting—such as lowering insulin and blood sugar—just as calorie restriction (fasting) does. This supplement is just one more option that can help support metabolic flexibility.

If you opt to try any of these supplements, I encourage you to have a conversation with your health care provider. Although these are supplements, they do have a powerful net impact on blood sugar, autophagy, etc.

Medicinal Mushrooms

Used for medicinal and food purposes for more than a thousand years, medicinal mushrooms have documented effects against different diseases, including infections and inflammatory disorders. A 2017 review in the *International Journal of Molecular Sciences* noted that: "Mushrooms are proven to possess anti-allergic, anti-cholesterol, anti-tumor, and anti-cancer properties."

Based on my study of medicinal mushrooms, I believe that their health benefits are amazing—which is why I recommend them as a complement to intermittent fasting. Medicinal mushrooms are high in antioxidants. They strengthen immunity and they stimulate autophagy. Among the most powerful medicinal mushrooms are: chaga mushrooms, cordyceps, reishi, turkey tail, lion's mane, and shiitake.

One of the most effective ways to use mushrooms during a fasted state is to add powdered forms to your coffee or green tea. As I noted above, they do not break your fast. Instead, you harness their health powers and support the healing that intermittent fasting is doing in your body. At the same time, they help prevent the overstimulating effects of caffeine.

Adaptogenic Herbs

These are naturally occurring plant compounds that can help support the brain and help with stress reduction, promote relaxation, and balance cortisol. These functions are very important while you're fasting, since fasting is a stressor.

There are many herbal adaptogens, but my favorites for use while fasting—and the best studied—are rhodiola rosea and ashwagandha.

The herb rhodiola has a long history of medicinal use in Russia, Scandinavia, and other parts of Europe. It is taken to boost energy, stamina, strength, and mental capacity; improve athletic performance; counter the effects of stress; and help manage depression and anxiety.

Clinical doses are commonly 200 to 600 milligrams daily.

Made from the root and berries of a small evergreen shrub grown in

India, the Middle East, and parts of Africa, ashwagandha contains chemicals that might help calm the brain, reduce inflammation, lower blood pressure, and enhance the immune system.

For stress, the suggested dosage is 300 milligrams, twice daily of the root extract.

Apple Cider Vinegar (ACV)

Apple cider vinegar, also sometimes referred to as ACV, is a vinegar made from fermented apple cider that offers a number of health benefits. For example, ACV can lower blood sugar and create more insulin sensitivity, both of which indirectly help promote fat-burning and support key reasons to fast. ACV can also increase feelings of fullness.

While fasting, use filtered ACV. If not fasting, you can consume raw unfiltered ACV. It contains proteins and bacteria, which can technically inhibit autophagy while you're fasting.

Some people like to dilute ACV in water and drink it down. Common dosages range from 1 to 2 teaspoons to 1 to 2 tablespoons daily mixed in a large glass of filtered water.

Detox Binders

These supplemental products assist your body in reducing its toxin levels by binding to and eliminating various toxins from your body. Although your body can do this on its own, sometimes the toxin load gets too high, and detoxification help is required. That's where detox binders come in. They work by:

- Eliminating toxic buildup
- Improving the lining of the gut
- Easing gas and bloating
- Absorbing poisons and preventing poisoning

If toxic overload is not corrected, toxins get recirculated back through organs, particularly the liver. This process puts an undue strain on your body as it tries to detoxify itself.

To support your body's detoxification pathways, I recommend a product called G.I. Detox. It contains several active ingredients:

- Zeolite clay. A clay formed from lava, it binds to and neutralizes toxins and is helpful in restoring gut microbial balance.
- Monomethylsilanetriol silica. This is made from silica, a naturally occurring substance found in the earth's crust, plants, and some vegetables. It detoxifies aluminum from the body and heals the gut lining.
- Humic and fulvic acid. Both are organic compounds from the earth that detoxify the body from herbicides and pesticides.
- Apple pectin. This is a type of fiber found naturally in apples that can improve gut health and help prevent or treat gastrointestinal and metabolic disorders.
- Activated bamboo charcoal. This fine black powder made from bamboo absorbs poisons from the body, including heavy metals. It also reduces intestinal gas and bloating.

Take one to two capsules a few times a week on an empty stomach. All binders should be taken either one hour before or two hours after medications and supplements. This timing prevents binding with the medication and supplements.

Supplements That Break Your Fast

Some supplements will hurt your fast, particularly anything with glucose or sugar in it, something that has more than 20 calories, or a supplement that should be taken with meals. Some of these might cause an increase in insulin, and this breaks your fast. Here is a list of supplements you should not take during your fasting window:

Any supplement you would normally take with meals, such as digestive enzymes, stomach acid and bile support products, fish oils, zinc, iron, and multivitamins/minerals (other than electrolytes). Others include:

- Branched-chain amino acids (BCAAs)
- Protein powder
- Creatine
- Fat-soluble vitamins (A, D, E, and K)
- Any herb that is required to be taken with food

Supplementing properly, plus maintaining a clean fast, is very beneficial to help you obtain all the benefits of fasting. I encourage you to keep your fasting time as pure as possible. Clear your mind, meditate, do yoga, stay hydrated, and appreciate all the positive effects taking place within your body and mind as you go through the next forty-five days.

To view the 16 references cited in this chapter,
please visit cynthiathurlow.com/references.

Chapter 8

· · · · · · · · · · · · · ·

Preparing for a Successful Fast

Now that you have a sense of what to eat, how to supplement, and what a fasting window looks like, you're about to start a new lifestyle of intermittent fasting. You'll ease into it with my IF:45 plan. Its gradual pace, geared to your life stage, helps your body adapt with a smoother transition and carries you over into an intermittent fasting lifestyle that will enhance your health over the long term.

There are different forms of intermittent fasting, but my plan primarily focuses on the 16:8 model (sixteen hours fasted, eight hours fed), also known as time-restricted feeding. If you're new to intermittent fasting, I recommend this model. It is an easy entry point into the intermittent fasting lifestyle and is easily adjustable to your schedule and daily habits. In my work with so many clients, I have found that the 16:8 model best supports weight loss and improves blood sugar, hormone balance, brain function, and longevity.

Intermittent fasting continues to be well researched. A study in 2020 in the journal *Cell Metabolism* found that this fasting method "resulted in weight loss, reduced abdominal fat, lower blood pressure and cholesterol." And, interestingly, the feeding window used in the study was 14:10 (fourteen hours fasted and ten hours feeding window), suggesting that a shorter fasting window works effectively, too.

Naturally, you want the best fasting experience possible and I hope after reading how beneficial it can be for your body that you're eager to give it a try! Yes, intermittent fasting is easier than many people initially think, but it is still a big change, and a few things need to be in order before you start. Jumping in too fast can sabotage the whole experience and leave you with a negative attitude toward fasting.

To make sure that doesn't happen, important factors need to be in play first. I see six criteria necessary in preparing for a successful fast.

1. Plan Your Fasting Schedule

Part of why the 16:8 model is so attractive and effective is because of its flexibility. Anyone, busy or not, can incorporate this model into their daily routine. It fits practically all lifestyles and gives concrete results, even with minimal effort. The key is to plan the fasting schedule that works best for you.

For starters, decide where to place your eight-hour eating window. Outside of that window, you consume no food for the other sixteen hours of each day. In practical terms, this is fairly easy since you will spend seven to eight of those hours asleep overnight. If you are sleeping, you are fasting! There are only a few hours of your waking days when you won't be eating and might feel a little hungry (although you become less hungry the more experienced you get at intermittent fasting).

Here is a typical daily picture of the 16:8 model. Let's suppose you set your feeding window between noon and 8:00 p.m. You'd get up in the morning, drink filtered water and tea (green or herbal tea) or coffee (but without milk or sugar) to help you wake up and put something in your stomach.

After waking up, you shouldn't really feel hungry. Our circadian rhythms dictate that ghrelin, the hunger-boosting hormone, is at its lowest in the morning, so you probably won't be hungry for at least the first few hours after you've woken up.

Then around noon, you'd have a meal. At about 7:30 p.m., it is time for dinner, and then you're finished eating until you start the entire schedule over again the next day.

In my typical feeding window, I follow a schedule similar to the one above—which gives me an eight-hour feeding window. You should do what works for you. Some people prefer one large meal and a snack; others want two meals. I suggest a bit of experimentation based on your own work and personal schedule. It is difficult to prescribe exactly when to eat, and what type of meal, because we are all bio-individual.

I usually break my fast around noon, although this varies based on my day. Sometimes it's earlier, sometimes it's later. My favorite go-to lunch is bacon and eggs tossed with vegetables or arugula with olives, extra-virgin olive oil, or avocado oil. Dinner tends to be mostly protein and non-starchy vegetables. My meals may not always be glamorous, but they meet my nutritional goals!

You can also ease into the 16:8 model by beginning with a larger eating window and then reducing it over time. For example, you could start by eating your first meal of the day by 9:00 a.m. and finishing your dinner at 9:00 p.m., a twelve-hour feeding window with a twelve-hour fast. Or: eat your first meal by 10:00 a.m. and finish your dinner at 8:00 p.m. with a fourteen-hour fast. Then transition to the 16:8 model.

If you're a morning person and doing 16:8, for instance, you might like an earlier schedule, breaking your fast with meal number one at 10:00 a.m. and closing the window at 6:00 p.m. Night owls who sleep in can try a 1:00 p.m. to 9:00 p.m. window.

Some women prefer a 9:00 a.m. to 5:00 p.m. eating window. This is great if you're a breakfast person. It gives you time for a solid breakfast in the morning, your regular lunch at noon, and an early dinner at 5:00 p.m., when your fast begins.

Or maybe you do shift work and are on the job overnight. That's fine. You can still fast when you're sleeping during the day and in the hours surrounding it. Fuel your body based on what works best for you. You can absolutely adjust your feeding and fasting windows around long shifts.

As you become more advanced as a faster, I'll show you how to shorten your eating window even more and increase your fasting hours.

There is no fixed schedule that is right for everyone so you're free to try out whatever time frame best suits you and your routine. Intermittent fasting works whatever your schedule, and regardless of when you open up your eating window. Remember that one key aspect of intermittent fasting is its *flexibility*.

2. Set Motivating Goals

Once you've decided on your fasting schedule, it's important to be clear about your fasting goals and what you want to achieve: Improved body composition? Weight loss? Weight maintenance? Improved metabolic flexibility? Reduced insulin or leptin resistance? Greater mental clarity? A physical and emotional detox? A resetting of poor eating and lifestyle habits? Antiaging?

In other words, why do you want to do intermittent fasting? Being crystal-clear about your goals anchors you while you're establishing this lifestyle. Goals give us purpose and direction and, like a compass, keep us headed in the right direction. The clearer you are of your motivations, the easier it will be. This principle applies not just to fasting but for everything else in your life, too.

I suggest writing your goals down in a journal, in your phone, or in your computer—somewhere you can see them or access them on a daily basis. Recording your goals helps increase your motivation for achieving your goals, makes them more concrete, and defines clearly what achieving those goals means to you. Studies have proven that people who write down their goals are 42 percent more likely to achieve them.

I am a big believer in manifesting, too, which is imagining everything you could ever want coming true by simulating the experience in your mind. You do this by visualizing what you want (your goal) and feeling what it's like to already have it.

When you actively visualize your ideal reality, something else amazing happens. You increase the neuroplasticity of your brain. Neuroplasticity is the brain's capacity to continue growing and evolving in response to life experiences, both real and *imagined*. Visualizing and manifesting thus have a rejuvenating effect on your brain.

When we visualize our desired outcome, we begin to "see" the possibility of achieving and having it. So—envision yourself already at your goal. To do this, create a detailed mental image of the desired outcome using all of your senses. Imagine how it feels physically in your body, emotionally, cognitively, energetically, and spiritually.

For example, if your goal is to lose fifteen pounds through intermittent fasting, visualize yourself at that weight—wearing a cute smaller dress or a bikini, moving with more confidence, feeling lots of energy, and so forth. Imagine the excitement, satisfaction, and thrill you will experience as you walk through life at a new, much healthier weight.

Keep visualizing and manifesting all the way to the achievement of your goals.

3. Change Your Limiting Beliefs

Limiting beliefs are long-held thoughts that hold us back and become barriers to success. Sometimes they are of our own making. Other times, they are implanted in our brains by others. A good example is when I was told: "Just accept your weight gain, you're getting older, and this is your life now." Because of such beliefs, we avoid doing certain things that could otherwise help us, which puts limits on our lives.

Here are some examples of common limiting beliefs around intermittent fasting and issues related to it:

It's impossible for me to go sixteen hours without food.
Fasting is not for me—I can't even last half a day without food!
I don't have the discipline to do intermittent fasting.
I feel weak if I go without food.

Wow, I could never do that.

Life ends after menopause.

I can't do anything about my hormones. I just have to accept that I'm aging.

Although these beliefs seem stuck in our gray matter, they are pretty easy to pry loose. The first step is to identify your own self-limiting beliefs—particularly about fasting and achieving your goals around it. Look over the list above. Can you relate to any of them? Which ones? Do you have others? Write them down and be honest when listing your beliefs.

Once you're finished, rank the beliefs in order, starting with the one that's holding you back the most. Which of your beliefs, if eliminated, would benefit you the most? How? Be specific in answering these questions.

Next, work on replacing your limiting beliefs with empowering ones. This is called "reframing" and involves asking yourself a few questions. Look at each belief and ask yourself: Is this really true? What evidence do I have to support this belief?

For example, let's say you believe the first one on the list: *It's impossible for me to go sixteen hours without food.* With some self-education and a little digging, you'll learn that an average person of normal body weight can subsist without food for forty days (more if you're heavier) and with all the nutrients and energy needed to survive. Thus, fasting should be generally safe, unless you fall into one of the categories of people who should not fast.

I'm not talking about forty days either—just twelve to sixteen hours, most of which take place overnight. Once you discover the falsehoods behind your limited belief, you've just refuted it, and you no longer need to hold on to it. Poof, it's gone.

Next, ask yourself: What are the consequences of this belief? Let's use the example of: *Life ends after menopause.* Consider the impact on your life if you hold on to this belief. For instance, you probably wouldn't pursue any positive life goals like traveling, starting a new business, running for office, or writing a novel. You wouldn't be improving your health for your later years.

Statistically speaking, women spend 40 percent of their lifetime in menopause, according to data from Simply Insurance. Let that sink in— that's nearly half your life! After menopause, the truth is that you have decades of amazing years left of great living! Start manifesting and visualizing how you'll use it, so that this belief does not become a self-fulfilling prophecy.

Finally, replace your limiting beliefs about intermittent fasting with ones that support your quest to improve your health and your life. For example, think to yourself:

> *It's easy for me to go sixteen hours without food because most of it will be overnight while I'm sleeping and I feel so amazing while fasting that it reinforces the health benefits of this lifestyle.*
> *Intermittent fasting will work for me because it has worked for so many others, and research supports its benefits.*
> *I have the discipline to do intermittent fasting. I will ease into it, one step at a time.*
> *I won't feel weak if I go without food because I will employ the strategies in this book.*
> *Wow, I can do this.*
> *Life begins after perimenopause and menopause. I have the freedom and time to achieve whatever I want.*
> *I can balance my hormones with natural strategies and put my body in reverse aging.*

Keep working on your list of limiting beliefs by replacing each one with a positive affirmation. Find any beliefs that do not serve you well and work to eliminate them using the steps I've laid out here. Do this on a regular basis, especially if you find yourself frustrated in any area of intermittent fasting.

Debunking the Top Five Intermittent Fasting Myths

Lots of myths about intermittent fasting are swirling around—and honestly, they fuel many of our self-limiting beliefs about fasting. These myths are misleading and create confusion about this important, life-changing strategy—which is why I want to blow the top myths out of the water. With the truth in hand, you're more likely to fast properly. And when you fast properly, you're more likely to experience all the benefits that intermittent fasting offers.

Myth #1: Intermittent fasting puts your body in a starvation mode.

Fact: This myth is probably one of the most common arguments against intermittent fasting. It is false. Fasting alters hormones that allow your body to tap into stores of food and nutrition for energy—namely, body fat and glycogen in your liver and muscles. After you eat, your body stores energy. If you don't eat (as in fasting), your body draws on that energy. There is no way intermittent fasting can lead to starvation because of this natural access of energy that goes on, day in and day out.

The other side to this myth has to do with the idea of starvation possibly causing a slower metabolism. This part of the myth leads people to believe that intermittent fasting will shut down the metabolism and prevent fat-burning. Totally untrue. In fact, intermittent fasts may increase your metabolic rate by drastically increasing blood levels of counter-regulatory, metabolism-stimulating hormones like norepinephrine. In fact, research reveals that fasting for up to forty-eight hours can boost metabolism by 3.6 to 14 percent. Metabolism is basically the process of turning food into fuel. So in effect, fasting leads to greater energy—which leads me to the next myth.

Myth #2: Intermittent fasting saps your energy.

Fact: You will not feel an energy drain when you intermittent fast—and here's why. When you fast intermittently, your insulin and glucose levels decrease, triggering your body to tap into an alternate energy source for fuel: body fat. In fact, many women report *higher* energy when they are in a fasting state. You'll actually feel more energized mentally, too. This is because intermittent fasting produces ketone bodies, which are by-products of fat-burning. And we know that specific types of ketones, such as beta-hydroxybutyrate (BHB), cross the blood-brain barrier to be used as energy. Remember: Your brain loves to run on ketones—and actually prefers them to glucose—so expect your concentration to sharpen and your brain fog to vanish with intermittent fasting. If you have less energy while fasting, it may be a sign that you are not properly fasting or it is not the right strategy for you.

Myth #3: Intermittent fasting makes you lose muscle.

Fact: Muscle tissue is important for weight control and health because it increases your metabolism. But some people believe that when you fast, your body starts burning muscle for fuel. The opposite is true: studies indicate that intermittent fasting is better for maintaining lean muscle. In one review, intermittent fasting caused a similar amount of weight loss as a calorie-restricted diet—but with much less reduction in muscle mass.

Remember, too, that intermittent fasting initiates surges in growth hormone, and this hormone supports muscle mass—so do not be too concerned about losing it when you fast. Those of us over age 40 may have to work a little harder for muscle, but it is not impossible.

Myth #4: Intermittent fasting causes food cravings.

Fact: The longer you practice intermittent fasting, the less hungry you'll feel.

Back when my life included three meals plus snacks in between, I was always hungry and fantasizing about my next meal. The desire to eat all day disappeared, along with the constant preoccupation with eating, after intermittent fasting became part of my lifestyle. So contrary to this myth, intermittent fasting liberates you from food cravings, as long as you are consuming adequate macros during your feeding window.

Studies consistently support the loss of cravings on fasting protocols. One was conducted in 2010 at the University of Illinois and involved people following an alternate-day fasting plan. It turned out that fasting did not increase their appetites. In fact, they ate 5 to 10 percent less than their "required" energy level on their eating days. Furthermore, the researchers concluded that people quickly adapt to fasting, and it blunts hunger, increases satisfaction, and sustains weight loss. You don't have to worry about cravings or an out-of-control appetite while fasting when you do it properly. Tip: If you do feel like your appetite is out of control or you have lots of cravings, you may need to break your fast earlier, although a shorter eating window is somewhat less effective.

Myth #5: Intermittent fasting is unsafe for women.

Fact: I really shake my head when I hear this one! In 2016, a research team published a review in the *Journal of Mid-Life Health* and enumerated a very long list of the benefits of intermittent fasting for women. The list blew me away. Intermittent fasting in women reduces body weight, controls blood sugar, slows tumor growth and reduces cancer risk, improves bone and joint health, protects the heart, improves mental health, and eases menopausal symptoms. All of these amazing benefits are directly attributable to the physiologic, metabolic, and hormonal processes I explained above. Intermittent fasting is a very powerful tool for women.

4. Enlist Social Support

Social support means having friends and family to turn to in times of need or for encouragement. Generally, social support enhances your quality of life and makes it easier to achieve your goals. Enlisting social support also helps boost your health. Researchers writing in the *European Journal of*

Clinical Nutrition, after reviewing the data on this subject, concluded: "Social support is important to achieve beneficial changes in risk factors for disease, such as overweight and obesity."

Thus, it is so important to have the right support system when starting a new diet or lifestyle. You need people to help you, encourage you, and promote your new journey to help your success.

Ideally, it's good to inform your loved ones and loop them in on the fact that you are starting an intermittent fasting program. Some people might not understand it—until you explain that most of it takes place overnight. It is also important to communicate why you're doing this—your goals—and how important it is to you to meet those goals. These days, fortunately, a lot of family and friends are fairly knowledgeable about healing methods like detoxing and fasting, so I doubt if you'll face any resistance. Plus, you'll usually be eating dinner, and dinner typically includes family. So your new program shouldn't create any big blips on the family radar.

There may be the occasional person who might be negative about your new journey. If so, it's best not to include them in your support circle.

If you're single, seek out "informational" social support. This involves finding as much positive information as you can on intermittent fasting—from books, articles, online sources, and studies, as well as talking to other people who successfully practice intermittent fasting.

My family is used to my intermittent fasting lifestyle, and your friends and loved ones will get used to it, too. In fact, I am fortunate enough to have a husband who will help batch-cook proteins and veggies for the week—which saves so much time. With our two growing boys we go through food quickly! So if you can, get family members in the act to support you. It helps to have help from a loved one who can watch out and care for you while you're fasting—and maybe even do it with you.

5. Get Healthy Sleep

As we get older, our daily need for quality sleep becomes more important than ever. As much as food is fuel for your body, so is sleep. It supports a healthy brain and endocrine system and balances all of your major hormones. You've got to get more deep sleep—especially if you want to be successful at intermittent fasting. One of my standard mantras is: If you cannot sleep through the night, please do not add intermittent fasting as a daily strategy.

Thus, you must work on sleep quality prior to starting my IF:45 plan. Fasting can be a stress to the body, and you will be negating any benefits if you are not sleeping properly.

Additionally, if you get fewer than six hours a night of sleep, your likelihood of becoming metabolically inflexible and insulin resistant increases substantially, and it becomes nearly impossible to lose weight without sufficient amounts of sleep. You will struggle with your cravings and with satiety, too. Getting both under control is vital for success with intermittent fasting.

Remember, too, that growth hormone is secreted at night while you're sleeping, and it is the hormone that is going to help your body heal and is key in terms of developing lean muscle mass. This secretion isn't going to happen unless you get into a deep sleep. If you are waking up between 2:00 and 4:00 a.m., you aren't getting into the deep sleep you need to lose weight, balance your hormones, and get the best from intermittent fasting. Waking up in this pattern is potentially indicative of poor blood sugar and hormone dysregulation.

Here are my guidelines for improving your sleep.

Sleep in a cold dark room (65 to 67 degrees). This mild drop in temperature induces sleep and affects the quality of REM (rapid eye movement) sleep, the stage in which you dream. Also, lower temperatures are conducive for hormonal regeneration overnight. Your bedroom also needs to be as dark as you can make it in order to encourage the secretion of melatonin. Purchase blackout curtains if needed. I also really like sleeping with a silk sleep mask.

Turn off electronics at least sixty to ninety minutes prior to bedtime. Computers, tablets, cell phones—all of these emit blue light, which interferes with melatonin production. If you can't avoid this, wear blue light–blocking glasses. They might not be the sexiest eyewear around, but they definitely help you sleep better.

Don't fall asleep with the television on. TVs also emit blue light. Plus, the television does not quiet your mind, it only excites it. Try going to sleep by reading a book, the old-fashioned kind with paper pages. This always works for me. Even better, don't have a TV in your bedroom. Your bedroom should be for sleep and sex—that's it.

Supplement with magnesium prior to bedtime. Our bodies use up this nutrient quickly as a way to combat stress. Having adequate magnesium levels helps your body slip gently into a restorative state. So as not to break your fast, use a pure magnesium oil spray that works transdermally.

Another option is to replenish your magnesium stores with a pre-bedtime foot soak or bath using Epsom salts. Add some lavender essential oils to further relax and calm yourself before bedtime.

Meditate. Meditation calms your brain down for better sleep. By definition, it is a mental exercise of emptying the mind and focusing on your breath. Try just taking deep breaths and focusing on your breath as an easy nighttime meditation. You'll be surprised at how quickly this technique can put you to sleep.

If you're new to meditation, try a guided meditation that takes you through it. Headspace offers a number of guided meditations that you can access through an app. Another mindful activity is to keep a gratitude journal, in which you record events and people in your life for which you are thankful. Reread each point, and meditate on what you've written.

Eat enough. Once you start intermittent fasting, don't drastically slash calories during your feeding window. The danger is that you'll get truly hungry, and hunger disrupts sleep. Your food choices during your feeding window should focus on protein and healthy fats. Adding in carbohydrates from starchy vegetables and low-glycemic fruits on higher carb days promotes restful sleep, too. Also, ensure that your feeding window closes three to four hours prior to bedtime in order to properly support your circadian rhythm.

Carve out a nightly ritual. This is one of my favorite ways to trick my brain into sleep because it helps support a healthy circadian rhythm. Determine what rituals work best for you and your lifestyle. Some ideas include: taking a hot bath before bedtime, going to bed around the same time every day, turning off the electronics, reading a book, and so forth. Do these every night so your body gets used to this routine and automatically starts relaxing in preparation for sleep.

Do a brain dump. Do you struggle with sleep because you have so many thoughts swirling around in your head? Buddhists describe this as our "monkey minds," referring to how our minds vault from thought to thought like monkeys swinging from branch to branch or tree to tree. If this process describes you, try a "brain dump." Grab a few blank sheets of paper and jot down everything that is on your mind. Then fold up your papers and put them aside. You've just released your worries, at least for the time being.

Don't drink alcohol prior to bedtime. Using a glass of wine or other alcoholic beverage to fall asleep is not ideal. Alcohol disrupts sleep, particularly REM sleep, more than almost anything else. It interferes with cortisol balance, increasing it at night when it should fall, and it suppresses melatonin production. If you do drink alcohol in the evening, follow it up with equal amounts of water and stick to your regular nightly ritual.

6. Establish a Stress Management Plan

No one lives a stress-free existence. I'm a realist and understand that we all need to find ways to address this proactively—especially women.

We are dealing with a lot of stressors, according to The Seattle Midlife Women's Health Study, a study spanning up to twenty-three years. As part of the study, eighty-one women responded to the question, "Since you have been in our study (since 1990 or 1991), what has been the most challenging part of life for you?"

The following aspects of midlife were listed as stressors:

Changing family relationships
Rebalancing work and personal life
Rediscovering self
Securing enough resources
Coping with multiple co-occurring stressors
Divorce or breaking up with a partner
Personal health problems
Death of parents

The enormity of stressors we face can keep us in a perpetual fight-or-flight situation with our sympathetic nervous system continually activated. Over time, this can wear our bodies down, elevate cortisol, and negatively impact our health. As I mentioned earlier, cortisol can cause us to gain weight, dysregulate insulin (another fat storage hormone), impact our immune function, and set in motion many other issues.

Remember that intermittent fasting is a stressor, so if you're persistently under stress, this is not the ideal time to fast. Work on reducing stress prior to starting the IF:45 plan. How you manage stress will be different from how I manage it, but here are some sustainable strategies proven to help.

Find exercises you enjoy.

Exercise is a wonderful stress reducer since feel-good chemicals called endorphins are released by your body when you exercise, also known as a "runner's high."

Please choose exercises you enjoy. Pushing yourself for the sake of exercising only creates more stress. Try walking, hiking, yoga, barre, solid core, cardio dance classes, swimming, paddle boarding, strength training, and so forth—whatever appeals the most to you and you feel like you can do it for a lifetime. (For more on exercising while fasting, see chapter 9.)

I prioritize moving my body every single day. I try to switch things up, as it's important to incorporate both higher intensity and active recovery exercises into your routine. I alternate between high intensity interval training (HIIT) and bodyweight exercises if working out at home, or lifting weights at the gym. Changing things up also prevents me from feeling bored with exercise.

Practice box breathing.
This is a form of meditation that greatly relieves stress. To do this: Exhale to a count of four and hold your lungs empty for another count of four. Inhale at the same pace, and hold air in your lungs for a count of four before exhaling and beginning the pattern anew.

Get grounded.
When was the last time you dug your toes in the sand or walked barefoot in the grass? I'm guessing it's been a while. If so, I highly suggest that you take your shoes off and just wiggle your toes in the lawn. This grounds you to Earth's natural energy and is immediately restorative to your system. You can lower your cortisol and increase your happy hormones, such as serotonin and dopamine, after a few minutes of letting your skin touch the earth.

Some twenty studies to date have reported that bodily contact with the Earth's natural electric charge stabilizes our physiology at the deepest levels; reduces inflammation, pain, and stress; improves blood flow, energy, and sleep; and generates greater well-being, according to a 2020 review published in the journal *Explore*.

Take a tech break.
Technology is a double-edged sword. On one hand, it enhances our lives in so many ways. If you've ever misplaced your cell phone or had your Internet go down for a few hours, you know what I mean. On the other hand, it can put us in a constant distracted state, in which we're always checking our email, texts, and social media accounts.

Social media, especially, is designed to be addictive. Research shows that when social media users receive positive feedback (likes), their brains fire off dopamine receptors—the same receptors involved in addiction to food, drugs, and alcohol. Dopamine is a reward chemical, released when we eat food that we crave or while we have sex, or when we check our social media, contributing to feelings of pleasure and satisfaction as part of the reward system. Not getting that dopamine surge from social media can add to personal stress.

My suggestion is to start incorporating tech breaks into your normal routine. No phone, no Apple Watch, no TV, no tablet. Nothing! Then observe the many independent, creative thoughts you have when not constantly distracted by technology. It's liberating, and you'll feel your stress levels dissipate.

Stay in the now.

Life unfolds in the present. But so often, we let the present slip away, as we worry about what may or may not happen in the future and regret what has passed.

One of life's greatest skills is the ability to pay attention to the present—staying in the now. This is all about mindfulness—seeing things as they are right this second, minute, or hour. It's about learning to enjoy, to relax, and to know the truth of where things are in your life. Rather than rush through your day, notice the little things—flowers blooming, farm animals with their babies, music in the air, and so forth. Become aware of your actions and your space. It leads to a greater sense of wonderment and joy. Mindfulness also reduces stress, boosts immune functioning, reduces chronic pain, lowers blood pressure, and generally helps us cope with tough issues in our lives.

Get some sunshine.

Enjoy fifteen to twenty minutes of sunshine daily (in the morning, preferably) so that your skin can properly manufacture vitamin D. Do not slather on sunscreen, either, for this short duration. It blocks the reaction between your skin and sunlight, which makes vitamin D. Going without sunglasses is important, too. It exposes our retina and our internal clocks to support healthy circadian rhythms and tells our bodies to get up and moving!

Adequate vitamin D from sunshine is a stress reliever because it helps your body make serotonin. Serotonin is associated with boosting your mood and helping you feel calm and focused. Vitamin D keeps you in balance, too, by preventing other types of hormonal deficits, including that of estrogen. Vitamin D also supports insulin sensitivity and a stronger immune system,

While you're outside allowing vitamin D to sustain your hormone levels, do other stress-relieving activities, such as playing with your pets, pulling weeds, gardening, or taking a stroll around the block.

Learn the power of no.
For an instant stress reliever, say "no" to requests when you have too much on your life plate or if you're cutting back on commitments. Overextending yourself is a huge stressor. "No" is a complete sentence, and you don't have to explain your reasons to anyone. Liberate yourself by saying "no" more often, and watch your stress levels improve.

Intermittent fasting can be a challenging adjustment period for your body, especially during the first few days. But by adequately preparing, you'll be less likely to quit and more likely to create a solid, lasting foundation for this amazing lifestyle.

To view the 13 references cited in this chapter,
please visit cynthiathurlow.com/references.

Part Three

Forty-five Days to Transformation

Chapter 9

· · · · · · · · · · · · ·

Phase 1: Induction—Days 1 to 7

Welcome to the Induction Phase!

Done properly, this phase jump-starts the IF:45 plan. The first seven days will help put your body into a state of ketosis in which it burns fat instead of glucose for energy. Your body will begin to feel the shift with initial weight loss, fewer cravings, and greater mental clarity as you acclimate to intermittent fasting. These early, positive results will motivate you, too, and inspire you to stay on track for the entire plan and beyond.

A lot can happen in just seven days. Catherine is a great example of what I hear early on from women who enroll in my IF:45 master class: "The biggest change I noticed the first week was that I had more energy and greater mental clarity. Also, I did not feel hungry—which was a pleasant surprise—and I did not have as many cravings for sugary foods like I used to have. I even dropped five pounds the first week! All of these benefits made me realize that I could make intermittent fasting a sustainable part of my lifestyle."

Detailing everything you need to be successful right away, this phase is full of practical tips on how to integrate intermittent fasting into your lifestyle and advice on how to make it go smoothly.

Remember, the IF:45 plan is not restrictive. But there are two very essential actions in this phase that will get you moving in the right direction: stop snacking and lower your carbohydrate intake.

Snacking, first of all, is counterproductive and has negative effects on your health and progress. Snacking:

- Spikes your blood sugar throughout the day, provoking higher insulin and ultimately fat storage. When you habitually snack, you cannot achieve metabolic flexibility. You also run the risk of developing insulin resistance.
- Prevents your body from burning fat for fuel. By contrast, with intermittent fasting, you train your body to tap into fat versus carbohydrates. Snacking interferes with this process.
- Creates inflammation. Eating triggers your immune system to produce a transient inflammatory response. And so if you eat around the clock, you can often end up in a near-constant inflammatory state. Snacking also causes gut microbes to leak into the bloodstream, silently triggering inflammation by the immune system.
- Interferes with the function of your migrating motor complex, or MMC. This key digestive system mechanism is the housekeeper of your small intestines and has an overall protective effect on your gut.
- Increases hormones, especially cortisol and insulin. High levels of both can cause those intense urges for sugar.

Also, the need to snack might indicate that your meals are improperly structured. But once you start organizing your meals around protein, fat, and fiber, you'll feel satiated, full of energy, and less likely to grab snacks. This mix of nutrients helps retrain your mind and body to not want to snack.

Remember, too, that one of the key principles of intermittent fasting is that you eat less often. Your blood sugar remains better balanced, which reduces insulin—and you burn fat, induce autophagy, and gain other benefits. It follows then that while fasting, you do not want to snack. Frequent snacking disrupts these benefits.

The second key principle of Induction is to follow a lower-carb eating plan, combined with intermittent fasting. Together, both help get your body into ketosis a bit faster. Ketosis is the metabolic state you reach when your body is breaking down fat as your primary fuel source and using ketones for energy. Ketones are the preferred method of fuel for the body.

On the IF:45 plan, you'll follow a nutrient-dense, whole-foods diet focused on protein, healthy fats, and fewer carbs. During Induction, the meal plans keep daily carbs at around 50 grams or less. At first, this is challenging for many people, especially if you have been consuming 200 to 300 grams of carbs daily. Slashing them by two-thirds will feel overwhelming at first. So I allow a little leeway: shoot for a range of 50 to 100 grams of carbs a day. After you get used to cutting carbs, you can lower them to 50 grams or fewer. Very important: Be sure to monitor your glucose and hunger cues as I explained on page 97. Everyone is different when it comes to carb intake, which is why I don't like to give blanket recommendations.

Besides jump-starting ketosis, lower-carb eating and intermittent fasting reduce inflammation, improve many health markers, and induce autophagy—that wonderful process in which dysfunctional and dying cells are replaced by new, healthy cells. Plus, you get other dual benefits: lowered insulin levels, lowered glycogen, satiety, greater energy, fat loss, and enhanced mitochondrial health.

Also, reducing your carb intake makes it easier to get through your fasting window. When you eat a diet focused on protein and on fiber with healthy fats and lower carbs, it becomes easier to fast without feeling hungry. Your body is fueling on its own stored fat, as well as on ketones. All of this helps create satiety.

A study in *PLOS ONE* suggests an additional reason you're less hungry on fewer carbs: hormones. Researchers compared blood tests of people who had eaten a high-carb meal with those who had eaten a high-fat or a high-protein meal. They found that the carb eaters had lower levels of the satiety hormones PYY and GLP-1 than the fat and protein eaters. Conversely, the fat and protein dieters had lower levels of the appetite-stimulating hormone ghrelin. So by lowering your carb intake, your hunger hormones are actively helping you stay satisfied for longer.

Other research shows that a low-carb diet is probably the most effective way to lose or maintain weight if you have insulin resistance or diabetes.

Fat Adaptation

Reducing carbs along with intermittent fasting also gets your body into "fat adaptation," in which you start using fat as fuel and not carbohydrates. Let me back up for a little metabolism 101. You can think of your metabolism like a campfire. If carbs burn hot and dirty like kindling, fats burn slowly and consistently like logs. Carbs are great for quick energy, but you don't want to be stuck in a carb-burning mode. In a carb-burning mode, you'd have to eat all day long (and become a slave to your snack stash) to keep your energy levels up (just as you have to keep feeding the fire with twigs). Ideally, you want your body to be able to switch into a fat-burning mode when needed—that's fat adaptation. Then you can easily go long stretches of time without needing food (because you can dip into your stored energy, aka body fat). Just as intermittent fasting helps your body transition into a fat-burning mode, so does a lower-carb diet.

This shift to fat adaptation usually begins over two to four days of eating 50 or fewer grams of carbs per day. But if you are slowly transitioning from a standard American diet with higher carbs, this process can take much longer, especially if you are stuck in a carb-burning mode. It might take your body a bit of time to "burn" through all the carbohydrate reserves in your liver. Think of this like training for a marathon. You have to start slowly and work up to burning higher amounts of fat. We are all different and bio-individual.

As you become more fat-adapted, you may notice an exciting benefit: the loss of inches from your body. Alison shared a photo of herself with the members of our recent master classes in which she was wearing a fitted sundress she had not worn in two years. Even back then, she had to put on shapewear to zip it up! After doing the IF:45 plan, Alison reported that although she had not dropped that many pounds, she was able to zip up the dress easily with room to spare. As Alison discovered, it's entirely possible to lose mostly body fat—which translates into inches—and not see much difference on the scale. Losing inches can be a sign that your body is burning fat and that you are more fat-adapted.

Diet Quality

While being lower in carbs, the meal plans in IF:45, including Induction, focus on diet quality—replacing refined carbohydrates with non-starchy vegetables, healthy fats, and quality protein. A November 2018 editorial in *Science* suggests that for most people, focusing on diet quality allows effective weight management and other benefits.

An important key to diet quality is to focus on eating "clean." This means getting most of your energy from protein and healthy whole-food fats like nuts and seeds, coconut, fish oils and animal fats, avocados, and olives and their oil.

Even though most of your calories will come from fat and protein, much of your plate should be taken up with non-starchy vegetables like leafy greens, broccoli, cauliflower, asparagus, zucchini, and cucumbers.

In contrast, stay away from processed, toxic seed oils. Instead, focus your attention on loading up on nutrient-dense veggies and quality fats and oils.

Supporting your body to depend less on carbs for fuel and more on fats and proteins for fuel will help you become more adept at fasting.

What to Expect During Induction

During Induction, your metabolism will shift as a result of fasting, reducing your carbohydrate intake, and increasing your fat intake. Instead of primarily using carbohydrates for energy, your body will start to switch to stored fat for fuel and changing it into ketones.

During this process, many people notice initial weight loss, but this is primarily due to losing the water that is stored in glycogen molecules in the liver. For every 1 gram of carbohydrate stored in the body as glycogen, there are approximately 2 to 3 grams of water stored. So when you first start a low-carb diet, the stored glycogen is released, along with the water that comes with it.

Other results you can expect from the Induction Phase:

- A loss of one to two pounds or more this week
- Fewer food cravings by the end of the week
- Improved digestion with less bloating and consistent bowel movements
- More energy
- Less brain fog

Each day, be sure to follow the meal plans that accompany the Induction Phase. See pages 215–216.

Day 1: Confirm your feeding/ fasting windows and stop snacking

To start out, it is a good idea to commit to your feeding/fasting schedule—and along with it, your morning routine. I covered much of this in chapter 7, but now it's time to get serious. For most people, the 16:8 model works best, or you can start with a twelve-hour fasting window and later extend it to sixteen hours.

Keep it simple. Think about it like this: There are two parts to your day—the fasting part and the eating part. So today, decide what time you're going to stop eating. Then you'll go to bed, wake up, and eat twelve to sixteen hours after you stopped eating. Part of the appeal of the IF:45 plan is that it is so easy, and you can adjust it to your lifestyle.

Also, establish your morning routine. This may involve having a cup of coffee or tea, along with a glass of water diluted with unflavored electrolytes. After I get dressed, I head to the kitchen and brew a cup of green tea for myself and my husband. I set out our supplements for the day. Then I'll drink my first glass of water with electrolytes (which I enjoy throughout the day).

On day 1, stop all snacking, too. Will you get hungry without snacks? It depends on our bio-individuality—some people might initially feel hungrier than others—and on our habits. Hunger can be a psychological habit. If your body is used to getting snacks at certain times, that's when it turns on the hunger signal. It's trying to sustain your ordinary, daily rhythm. This can be a sign that you need to adjust your macros, mainly protein or fat or a combo of each to reach the point where you are not getting hungry in between meals.

But the good news is when you alter that rhythm, when you break your snacking habits, your body quickly adapts to the new daily cycle. For most women, it only takes two or three days for the body to adjust to the new routine. Your body then starts turning off those snack signals.

So what can you do in the meantime? A couple of suggestions:

STAY HYDRATED. Drink water with electrolytes during the times you are not eating while you're adjusting to the routine. This can help you stay full. Most of us don't drink enough water, anyway. Signals of hunger can actually be a sign that you're thirsty. Drink up to half your body weight in ounces of water daily, supplemented with electrolytes.

INCLUDE OTHER FLUIDS. These are coffee and herbal teas, without sweeteners, milk, cream, or creamers. Their flavors inform the body that food is incoming, and then the body prepares hormonally for the digestion process. This just makes fasting harder.

INCREASE THE AMOUNT OF HEALTHY FATS YOU HAVE AT MEALTIME. They play a huge role in creating a feeling of satiety that lasts until your next meal. See page 98 for my discussion of healthy fats.

SALT YOUR FOOD. I love Redmond's products for this purpose. Another good salt is red salt. Less processed than most salts, red salt contains pure trace minerals and is sourced from natural origins. Other good choices are Celtic sea salt and Himalayan pink salt, both of which provide minerals and trace minerals. It is amazing how satiating adding the right salt is to your meals and it helps with electrolytes, too!

By contrast, processed salt contains synthetic iodine, anticaking substances, bleaching agents, residues, and other artificial additives. Just as you should avoid refined flour or refined sugar, stay away from processed salt.

Day 2: Do a kitchen clean-out

Today's action item is to do a pantry clean-out. Being successful with fasting goes hand in hand with good nutrition, so look in your pantry, fridge, and freezer and get rid of all high-carb, sugary products that might be consumed in a moment of weakness. Eliminate any temptation. Give these foods away, toss them out, or donate them.

Here is a sample list of items to eliminate:

Pantry
Candy
Cake mixes, including pancake mixes
Cookies
Crackers
Breads
Bagels
Sugar in all forms, including syrups and honey
White and whole-wheat flours
Gluten-containing carbs, including grains
Muffins
Breakfast cereals
Pasta
Rice
Potato chips and other processed snack foods
Popcorn
Dried fruits

Canned soups
Canned fruit
Seed oils

Fridge
Soft drinks and fruit juices
Applesauce
Fruits, except berries
Jams
Margarine
Everything that says "low fat" or "no fat"
Condiments that list "sugar" in the top four ingredients
Dairy foods (cheeses, milk, etc.)
Potatoes and other starchy vegetables

Freezer
Ice cream
Frozen desserts
Frozen bread products
Cakes
Ready-made or toaster waffles or pancakes
Frozen fruits, except unsweetened berries
Pizza

With your kitchen clean-out done, here's a look at how to restock it for the IF:45 plan. The following foods will optimize your results by keeping glucose and insulin steady and kicking you into ketosis. Get familiar with the foods on the list and work them into your lifestyle.

EGGS—Look for organic and free-range or pastured.

MEAT AND POULTRY—Select organic, grass-fed meats and don't overdo processed meats like bacon and salami.

FISH AND SEAFOOD—Shop for wild-caught fish, such as salmon, tuna, sardines, shrimp, scallops, mahi mahi, and cod. (Avoid eating predatory fish like shark, swordfish, king mackerel, or tilefish because they contain high levels of mercury.)

Low-carb vegetables—Load up on veggies such as asparagus, artichokes, leafy greens, zucchini, green beans, peppers, onion, garlic, mushrooms, summer squash, and especially detoxifying cruciferous veggies such as broccoli, cauliflower, Brussels sprouts, bok choy, and so forth. Also, look for veggies rich in deep pigmentation.

Fresh herbs—Get parsley, cilantro, rosemary, thyme, dill, chives, and green onions.

Low-sugar fruits—Stock up on berries in small quantities (strawberries, blueberries, raspberries, mulberries, blackberries, and cranberries); lemons and limes; apricots, cherries, nectarines, peaches, and plums; and tart apples.

Condiments—Get coconut aminos (a soy-free soy sauce replacement), fish sauce, Cholula hot sauce, organic tahini, and any condiment in which sugar is not among the top four ingredients.

Healthy fats—Look for extra-virgin olive oil, olives, coconut oil, coconut cream, C8 MCT oil, avocado oil, avocados, nuts, seeds, grass-fed butter, ghee, lard, duck fat, and tallow; nut milks without additives such as the Malk brand. Nuts and seeds are calorically dense and easy to overeat, so keep your portions small.

Other items—Get almond flour, canned coconut milk, bone broth, coffee, and teas (opt for organic).

Supplements—Decide on which supplements you want to take based on the information in chapter 7.

Foods, Herbs, and Spices That Trigger Autophagy

Autophagy is stimulated when you fast. It kicks in more rapidly if you're already in a state of ketosis, and sometimes it starts working in as little as twelve hours, especially when you combine a high-fat, low-carb diet with intermittent fasting.

Autophagy boosters include:

- Cacao
- Cinnamon
- Coffee
- Curcumin (found in the spice turmeric)
- Ginger
- Green tea
- MCT oil, predominately formulated with C8 fatty acids
- Mushrooms
- Organic olive oil
- Resveratrol—a powerful plant compound that can be found in red wine, grapes, berries, and peanuts

Day 3: Develop a meal prep habit

Meal prepping is a great habit to develop on the IF:45 plan. It saves time by getting things ready ahead of time. In fact, one study published in the *American Journal of Preventive Medicine* suggests that spending time on preparing and cooking meals at home is linked with better dietary habits.

I always like to have prepped ground beef, pulled chicken, and hard-boiled eggs in my fridge in case I need to create a quick meal. I also like having veggies precut and roasted. I do my meal prep on Sunday and Wednesday. That's when I put together a bunch of meals that my family and I can warm up throughout the week. And I prep a lot of food, because I have teenage boys, and they eat a ton of food.

There are lots of ways to go about your own meal prep, but here are a few ideas to get you started:

PICK ONE OR TWO DAYS PER WEEK TO DO ALL THE WORK. Select your prep day or days when you devote time to preparing meals. After that, you will have most of the work done for the entire week!

DOUBLE UP. Prepare doubles of some of your favorite recipes each time you make them. Save the leftovers for another meal to freeze for later.

HARD-BOIL EGGS AND STORE THEM IN YOUR FRIDGE. Eggs are an excellent source of protein, vitamins A and B, and healthy fat—perfect on a low-carb diet.

CHOP OR SPIRALIZE RAW VEGETABLES IN ADVANCE. Then store them in baggies or containers in your fridge. Cutting veggies in bulk saves lots of precious time.

ROAST DIFFERENT VEGETABLES WITH THE SAME COOKING TIME. I love roasted veggies because roasting brings out their natural sweetness. But waiting for them to cook can be time-consuming around dinnertime. To prep a large batch of veggies, roast them together, based on their roasting time. Bake faster-cooking vegetables such as asparagus, mushrooms, and cherry tomatoes in the same pan; and bake slow-roasting vegetables like carrots, cauliflower, and onions together.

BAG UP SMOOTHIE INGREDIENTS. If you like smoothies, save yourself time by pre-assembling and freezing the ingredients. Measure out your berries and your greens, then bag them and place them in the freezer.

MAKE SALAD JARS FOR LUNCH. Place your dressing in the bottom of a mason jar, layer sturdier veggies like cucumbers and peppers on next, followed by leafy greens. Put a paper towel square on top (this keeps leafy greens fresh and crisp), and screw on the lid. No more soggy salads for lunch.

PRECOOK PROTEINS. Poultry, fish, and meats—virtually any proteins—can be cooked ahead of time, then heated up when you're ready to enjoy them.

Day 4: Get physical activity every day

If you haven't already, establish a daily exercise activity. Yes, you can work out while fasting—and you should—because it can help speed up your transformation.

Many fasters, including me, exercise in the morning. If they are following the 16:8 model, their workouts fall within the fasted time frame, and that's very effective. Working out during the fasting period means you'll use more of your stored fat for energy. Plus, your muscles will be primed by your workout so they can better absorb proteins and nutrients after you break your fast with your first meal of the day.

There are other benefits, too. Any kind of exercise is known to increase insulin sensitivity, which means that your body will use insulin more efficiently. Research has also found that working out while fasting can increase growth hormone, that antiaging chemical that is so crucial for maintaining and building muscle.

To maintain a successful fast while working out, here are a few important tactics to consider.

STAY HYDRATED. Purified water and herbal teas throughout the previous day and early morning are essential for a successful fast and productive workouts. Also, if you want to properly prep your muscles, have some water forty-five to sixty minutes before you work out. Don't forget electrolytes!

DON'T SKIP DINNER. When creating your morning workout schedule, make sure that you ate dinner the night before. If you have a tendency to skip dinner, you won't have enough of the fuel or energy that you need. When you eat, have a balanced plate of protein, healthy fat, and vegetables.

LISTEN TO YOUR BODY. Even once you've adapted to combining intermittent fasting and exercise, stay alert to how your body is responding day to day. If it feels like too much, or you feel like you're running out of gas, it's best to slow down. Do some more gentle workouts such as yoga or walking.

TIME YOUR MEALS AND EXERCISE. You no longer have to worry about eating before a workout once you are fat adapted; you can go to the gym, lift weights, and then break your fast at your normal time. In fact, most women will state that they feel 100 percent better working out fasted than dealing with food sloshing around in their digestive tract.

DON'T WORRY ABOUT POST-WORKOUT SUPPLEMENTS OR MEALS. A lot of misinformation is circulating about this issue. The truth is, you don't need supplements after a workout—especially BCAAs or protein shakes—unless you are perhaps a competitive bodybuilder preparing for a contest. If you work out at 6:00 a.m., your blood sugar and muscle tissue repair will be fine by 10:00 a.m., when you are ready to break your fast. Developing muscle, losing body fat, and maintaining balanced blood sugar are more about consistent, quality macros over time. If you follow my intermittent fasting advice and are already eating whole foods, your body will reap the benefits of a good sweat session. The best pre-workout beverage can be plain coffee or herbal tea.

CHEW YOUR FOOD. Chewing your food thoroughly allows your body to absorb as many nutrients as possible. Whole, chewable food is always superior to drinking a protein shake. I don't care how clean your protein powder is, it is still processed. Also, the brain registers satiety when you chew. Keep in mind that the digestive process starts in your brain. You can't be stressed out and properly digest your food at the same time. Being in a relaxed state of mind helps aid digestion!

WATCH WHERE YOU ARE IN YOUR MENSTRUAL CYCLE. If you are still in your cycling years, avoid strenuous exercise and fasting the five to seven days prior to your menstrual cycle.

With these tactics in mind, there are some situations in which people should not work out in a fasted state. If you are a sugar-burner (which means you primarily burn carbs—sugar—for energy) and have hypoglycemia, you probably won't feel good exercising while fasted. Sugar burners feel like they need to snack around the clock, they have trouble feeling satiated after meals, and they crave sweets and carb-rich foods. (See below for more information on sugar burners.)

Otherwise, most people can exercise while fasting because they have become fat-adapted—their bodies are burning fat and not burning sugar. While working out fasted, you should feel like this: Your energy is stable; your mind is clear; you feel good; and you're not hungry, queasy, or shaky.

Day 5: Get fat-adapted more quickly

If you have habitually eaten a lot of processed carbs in the past, you are probably a sugar burner. Metabolically, your glucose and insulin levels are dysregulated. When you start intermittent fasting, there is a time lag as your body reluctantly turns from burning the quick energy of glucose to harvesting fuel from your fat stores. So naturally, you want to do whatever you can to become more fat-adapted. That way, you're better able to burn your stored body fat for energy. It also reduces your body's cravings for carbs. You may also feel more full after meals, resulting in eating fewer calories throughout the day and leading to weight loss.

Here are my strategies to help you become more easily fat adapted, in addition to fasting and reducing your daily carbohydrate intake.

EAT MORE FAT. As you decrease your carbs, you'll want to increase your intake of dietary fat. Eating fat can help train your cells to run on fat. That said, fat is more calorically dense (9 calories per gram) than protein or carbohydrates (both 4 calories per gram), so if you eat a high-fat diet, you may need to eat smaller portions. Examples of proper portion control include ¼ avocado, ¼ cup of nuts, or 1 tablespoon each of olive oil, coconut oil, butter, or ghee.

How much fat should you have daily? It depends on how much weight you are trying to lose or how metabolically flexible you are. If your goal is weight loss, you might want to limit your fat intake to one or two servings per meal. If you are metabolically flexible, and you burn fat efficiently, you can probably handle more servings of fat a day. Make sure you choose high-quality fats.

Also, dietary fat has a much smaller impact on insulin levels than carbs do. This low-insulin state helps you stay in fat-burning, not fat-storage, mode. In your quest for fat adaptation, you should eat lots of healthy fats like those listed above.

INCLUDE C8 MCT OIL. Medium-chain triglycerides (MCTs) contain fatty acids that have a chain length of six to twelve carbon atoms. They are important fat burners since they circumvent the usual digestion of fat.

They go right away to the liver and facilitate the production of ketones. The body starts using ketones for energy. Your cells then get accustomed and adapted to using ketones as fuel and become more efficient at it.

There are four main types of fatty acids in MCTs: caproic acid (C6), caprylic acid (C8), capric acid (C10), and lauric acid (C12). If you don't mind paying a little extra, purchase a C8 MCT oil. Its benefits over the others are that it:

- Boosts metabolism
- Increases fat adaptation
- Reduces hunger by raising the hormone leptin and PPY, both of which reduce the hunger hormone ghrelin
- Improves insulin sensitivity
- Fuels the brain
- Provides almost instant energy

In some people, MCT oil can initially be a little irritating to the digestive system, causing loose stools and diarrhea. So start slowly by using 1 teaspoon at a time and gradually increasing your dosage. It can be put in coffee, used in salad dressings, and drizzled over vegetables. The MCT oil I recommend is my Simply Energy.

MONITOR YOUR GLUCOSE STABILITY. Use your continuous glucose monitor or glucometer to check blood sugar, response to carbohydrate intake, and hunger cues.

WORK OUT IN A FASTED STATE. This enhances your fat utilization and decreases your reliance on outside fuel sources like carbs for energy. Your fat adaptation will progress and stabilize. Fasting and exercise are a great combination for fat adaptation. (See my tips above for how to exercise successfully when you're fasting.)

Day 6: Try going grain-free

Eating gluten-free and grain-free foods involves avoiding not only wheat products containing gluten but also any gluten-free grains, such as rice, corn, oats, millet, amaranth, and so forth. There are recognized benefits of going grain-free.

For one thing, it helps curb carb addictions. Most grains can trigger a big increase in glucose—which makes you want to eat even more grains. When you get off grains, you can help avoid this addictive response.

Also, many grains are sprayed with dangerous pesticides and chemicals. A paper published in *Interdisciplinary Toxicology* suggested that Monsanto's glyphosate (in Roundup) may directly cause the development of celiac disease (an autoimmune disease in which people cannot eat gluten).

An equally serious issue is that glyphosate usage is one of the main reasons gluten today is so toxic. In the United States, a common farming practice with wheat is to drench the wheat fields with Roundup several days prior to the harvesting in order to produce a larger yield. The glyphosate in Roundup significantly disrupts the functioning of our microbiome and contributes to hyper-permeability of the intestinal wall (leaky gut syndrome), resulting in potential autoimmune disease symptoms. Eating contaminated grains may thus make you susceptible to autoimmune disorders such as celiac disease and others.

There is also some evidence that eliminating grains can help lower cholesterol and LDL (not-so-good cholesterol), and has a huge impact on reducing triglyceride levels.

What's more, a diet free from gluten and grains has been shown to improve anxiety and depression, often seen in perimenopausal and menopausal women.

I recommend to many of my patients and clients that they eliminate gluten and grains for six weeks. There are other benefits for doing so, besides preventing autoimmune diseases. Eating grain-free can potentially help improve food sensitivities, thyroid problems, fatigue, headaches, skin issues, and weight gain.

Trust me, you won't miss grains as much after you discover and start eating some delicious grain substitutes, such as:

- Cauliflower rice
- Shirataki noodles (much like tofu, these noodles pick up the flavor they are cooked with)
- Cabbage rice
- Spiralized vegetables such as zucchini (zoodles)
- Spaghetti squash
- Portobello mushroom (a great alternative to burger buns)
- Lettuce wraps
- Cauliflower pizza crust
- Zucchini lasagna (thinly sliced zucchini cut lengthwise as an alternative to lasagna noodles)

Day 7: Be inspired

Stay in the right mindset. Review your goals and congratulate yourself on your progress. Make sure limiting beliefs don't slip back into your thoughts. Think empowering thoughts instead, and keep them simple like: *I know intermittent fasting is good for my health. I love the results so far. I can keep going. My body is responding, and it's amazing.*

Consider writing your thoughts and goals down and keeping them in a prominent place so that you stay in the right mindset throughout the IF:45 plan.

Studies prove that motivation starts the action, but the daily habits will ensure you get closer to your goals.

It is always a good idea to journal your fasting experience, too. Journaling helps you identify triggers, record progress, and celebrate triumphs. You can also write down your favorite meals, recipes, and exercise plans.

Here is a sample journal entry from one of my IF:45 fasters who reflected on her experience:

Intermittent fasting has helped me simplify my decision-making around food. After a 16-hour fast, I am very conscious about what I break the fast with. I enjoy the discipline of the fasting process as well—just what I needed after so many unsuccessful attempts with diets. Life is changing for me. I think more clearly. I am at peace with my body. My waistline is smaller. Intermittent fasting is my new norm. I'm so very thankful.

To view the 17 references cited in this chapter,
please visit cynthiathurlow.com/references.

Chapter 10

Phase 2: Optimization—Days 8 to 37

You've had one week of cleaning up your diet and your kitchen. You've stopped snacking, reduced carbohydrates, and set the stage for becoming fat adapted. Now you're ready to commit to thirty more days of living a health and wellness lifestyle, backed up by intermittent fasting.

In this phase, we're going to change things up a bit. You'll increase your carbohydrate intake to a more moderate level, focus on carb cycling, and customize your fasting and feeding window to your stage in life.

Like last week, I'll continue to guide you daily with additional guidelines and strategies so that you can continue your success on my IF:45 plan.

What to Expect on Optimization

As you move through Optimization, you'll feel even more positive effects of intermittent fasting and lower-carb eating—such as improved mental clarity and more energy. Although everyone is different, by the midpoint of Optimization, your body will have accomplished most of its work in adapting to using fat for energy. Also, your hunger and food cravings will be mostly diminished, and your stamina and vitality will be higher.

All of these benefits came true for Anne, a participant in one of my recent master classes. Toward the end of Optimization, she had this feed-back to share: "I'm excited that I feel much better. I have energy and mental clarity like never before. I no longer crave junk food. Nor do I have the desire to snack between meals. I have lost seven pounds—something I could not do even when I was working out six days a week. My hot flashes are less frequent too. I'm excited to keep pressing forward on this journey—for a lifetime."

Like Anne, you can expect some gratifying benefits from this phase. For example:

- Greater mental clarity
- Increased autophagy
- Reduction in insulin levels
- Weight loss
- Improved digestive health and rest
- Better sleep quality

As with the first seven days, let's jump into Optimization with day-by-day strategies to help you succeed. Be sure to follow the daily Optimization meal plans, beginning on page 217, for the next thirty days.

Day 8: Increase your water intake with electrolytes

Water is a big player when it comes to successful intermittent fasting, so let's up your game here. Commit to drinking half your body weight in ounces of water daily. Water aids in digestion and helps you stay hydrated throughout the day. Filtered water is best, and don't forget your electrolytes (see chapter 7 for more information on electrolytes).

Sometimes it is helpful to have a visual aid to encourage and remind you to drink up. I keep a stainless steel or glass water bottle nearby to remind me of how much water to drink.

Day 9: Understand what to eat after your daily fasting window ends

When it's time for your first meal after you've fasted, fuel up on the right foods—protein, healthy fats, and non-starchy vegetables. This mix is satiating and more likely to hold you over to your next meal, while dishes heavy on refined carbs and sugar will leave you feeling hungry again relatively quickly because they spike glucose and insulin.

Some people prefer to have a light meal like salad, non-dairy yogurt with a few macadamia nuts and berries, or even bone broth. Experiment to find what works best for you.

Lately, I have been eating a small beef grass-fed burger with kale and cashew pesto, but the options are endless: bone broth, jicama and raw veggies with clean hummus, nut butters, or a salad with protein and healthy fats. You want a whole-foods diet with as many unprocessed foods as possible. The meal plans for Optimization will help you plan.

Day 10: Resolve elimination issues

Many Americans and people of most first-world countries struggle with proper digestion and elimination. Our foods are so processed, void of natural fiber, that our exposure to good bacteria has also dwindled, and we struggle with constipation. Other causes are lifestyle issues such as low physical activity, stress, and lack of relaxation. All of these can be aggravated by an underactive thyroid, underlying food sensitivities, dehydration, dysbiosis, and often certain medications such as antidepressants, blood pressure medication, and drugs for acid reflux. If you're experiencing these issues:

- Increase your water intake and supplement with electrolytes (see chapter 7).

- Eat more fiber-dense foods, especially apples, figs, prunes, and cruciferous veggies (broccoli, Brussels sprouts, cauliflower, and so forth).
- Move your body daily.
- Work on stress. You must be relaxed to "go" and in the right frame of mind. This is because digestive issues are under the control of your parasympathetic nervous system, which governs rest and relaxation.
- Add in bile-supportive foods: beets, artichoke hearts, and sauerkraut.
- Eat 1 tablespoon daily of fresh ground chia seeds and flaxseeds during your feeding window (seeds will break a fast); sprinkle them on a salad or toss them into a smoothie.
- Have two green salads daily.
- Consider supplementing with hydrochloric acid (HCl) and digestive enzymes. See the Best Practices section for suggested products.
- Use food sensitivity testing to help determine foods that may be contributing to constipation.
- Have your thyroid checked through blood tests.
- In some instances, magnesium supplements, especially magnesium glycinate, can help gently move the bowels.
- Occasionally sip Smooth Move Tea—but not every day because it contains the herb senna, which in excess amounts can irritate the gut.
- Add probiotics, including probiotic-rich foods (kefir, kombucha, and fermented veggies) into your diet daily.

Day 11: Do a vegetable juice fast today

Surprising your system with a change in what you're eating can help keep things interesting—which is why I suggest a vegetable juice fast once a month. I have done this for the past two years. Initially, I was very skeptical.

But, after several times, I now look forward to it each month. I have found that making it to 24+ hours has become easier and easier each time.

During a juice fast, you consume primarily vegetable-based juices—three to six 8-ounce servings. Do this within your feeding window, too, in order to preserve your fasting schedule.

Juice has no fiber. But the temporary absence of fiber gives your digestive system a rest. Your body can then easily assimilate key vitamins and minerals that may be missing from your diet.

The research on the benefits is ongoing, but there is data to suggest that juice fasts have a favorable impact on the gut microbiome and overall health. A 2017 study published in *Scientific Reports* noted that vegetable juice is an excellent source of "prebiotics," which are essentially food substances that healthy gut bacteria feed on, as well as polyphenols, beneficial plant compounds thought to boost digestion and brain health and protect against heart disease, type 2 diabetes, and even certain cancers. To analyze the possible benefits of a juice fast, the researchers tested twenty healthy adults who consumed only vegetable/fruit juices for three days. During that time, the juice-based diet altered the gut bacteria associated with weight loss, raised levels of nitric oxide (a substance that helps open up blood vessels), and decreased free radical activity.

The Health Benefits of a Vegetable Juice Fast

Lowered body fat
Healthier microbiome
Reduced incidence of cancer
Improved immune function
Slowed bone loss
Reduced risk of diabetes and cardiovascular disease
Antiaging

Before you take part in this juice cleanse, be aware that not all juices are created equal. Choose a high-quality juice that is:

- Raw and alive—not treated with pasteurization or high-pressure processing (HPP), both of which destroy the intrinsic nature of the vegetables
- Cold pressed (protects the enzymes from oxidation)
- Prepared from mostly vegetables and very little fruit
- Created from organic produce

You can find a juice company that fills the requirements mentioned above, or you can create juices yourself with a good juicer. If you prefer to not make your own, two sources I recommend are Farmers Juice and The Weekly Juicery (see Best Practices, in the Appendix, for more information).

Be sure to drink your juice on an empty stomach. This helps extend digestive rest, which is very beneficial for your gut.

Day 12: Lower your carb grams

This recommendation is for non-cycling women: Up until now, you may have been sticking to a carb range of 50 to 100 grams daily. If so, consider reducing this to 50 grams daily, or slightly below.

Try this and see how you feel. You may have to adjust down or up because everyone is different. You'll know if you've hit the right intake if you feel satiated and have improved mental and physical energy throughout the day.

Day 13: Introduce carb cycling and adjust your IF schedule to your cycle

If you are cycling, follow your regular fasting and lower-carb lifestyle up until five to seven days preceding your menstrual cycle. These days, you will shorten your fasting window to twelve to thirteen hours and consume larger portions of healthy, quality carbohydrates. Examples include root vegetables like beets, carrots, parsnips, rutabaga, sweet potatoes, turnips, and yams. Winter squashes are also good choices, as are low-sugar fruits like berries. You have increased insulin sensitivity during this time period. These foods will help reduce cravings and provide optimal hormone support. See the chart below for exact recommendations on how to carb cycle.

If you should notice changes in your menstrual cycle, be sure to:

- Recognize that your cycle may be impacted for one or two cycles (longer, shorter, lighter, or heavier periods). If your period goes away, that's a different issue. I truly believe that our menstrual cycles are a vital sign and must be taken very seriously. Therefore, if your cycle stays inconsistent or goes away, it is a sign that you need to take a break from fasting and/or also see your health care provider.
- Increase your hydration and make sure you are supplementing with electrolytes (see chapter 7)
- Adjust your macros
- Work on sleep quality and stress management
- Scale back on your exercise intensity
- Stop fasting for a while until your cycle normalizes
- See your health care provider for a checkup and lab tests

If you are no longer cycling, you can stick to the 16:8 model. Later in this phase, I will show you how to extend your fast.

Day 14: Prepare for the weekend

The weekend often throws off our weekday feeding and fasting schedule, but that's fine because the IF:45 plan is so flexible. For example, if having a Sunday brunch with your family is a high priority, shift your feeding window to accommodate this. If you go out to dinner on a weekend night, and this is important to you, adjust your feeding window accordingly.

The IF:45 plan is actually one of the easiest programs to stick to while enjoying nights out because you can change your fasting window to accommodate special events and family dinners. All you need to do is position your feeding window for when you want to go out, whether for a lunch date or for dinner. I want you to get into the mindset that you can have fun and still do support practices that impact your long-term health.

Day 15: Rethink your hunger cues

Often, when you think you feel hungry, it's not necessarily true physiological (body) hunger but rather psychological (emotional) hunger. Once you realize this, then all it takes is a little bit of patience as your body adjusts to the IF:45 plan. Here are some guidelines for managing hunger that you can put in place today.

EMPHASIZE PROTEIN AND FAT. Protein stimulates hormones that tell your body and brain you've eaten enough. Fat is gratifying and satiating and has been shown to reduce calorie and food intake at meals.

DON'T MISTAKE HUNGER FOR DEHYDRATION. Hunger signals can be misleading. Oftentimes, you just need more water.

BREW SOME GREEN OR HERBAL TEA OR COFFEE. These help suppress your appetite and help to reduce hunger.

STAY BUSY. Distraction is a wonderful thing! So, structure your fasting hours around activities when you can.

PRACTICE MINDFULNESS. This is an excellent way to combat emotional eating, when you feel hungry out of boredom, loneliness, depression, or anxiety. Each time you hear yourself say, "I'm hungry," ask yourself if you're bored, stressed, anxious, sad, or tired instead. Then mindfully meditate on the positive changes taking place in your body, or on your goals and how you will feel after you achieve them.

Day 16: Ease detoxification side effects

As your body detoxes from processed carbs and toxins, you may experience some side effects, such as headaches, dizziness, or nausea (the typical "keto flu" symptoms mentioned earlier). At first, you might feel alarmed by these, but there's no need to worry. The side effects are actually positive signs that your body is returning to a state of health.

But often, these side effects can be related to poor hydration and lack of electrolytes. Low blood sugar, low sodium, and lack of exercise are also triggers. Some people get these side effects from transitioning too quickly from eating mini-meals and snacks to a feeding window of two daily meals.

The body also stores toxins in fat tissue to keep them from doing system-wide damage. So when you lose weight, you're releasing some of these stored toxins into your bloodstream. If your detoxification pathways are not adequately open (stool, urine, breathing, sweating, and so forth), there can be a slowdown of detoxification processes, and this also leads to side effects.

While your body is adjusting, it is a good idea to minimize these side effects. Here's how.

- Get adequate hydration with electrolytes (see chapter 7)
- Make sure you're not snacking and build your main meals with protein and healthy fats
- Move your body daily and get adequate rest
- Try infrared saunas to promote detoxification
- Supplement with the binder G.I. Detox to support elimination and detoxification. Be sure to take these at least one hour before or two hours after other supplements and medications.

Day 17: Get back into ketosis after the weekend

Maybe you ate too much over the weekend or didn't stick fully to your fasting/feeding schedule. First of all, forgive yourself. Feeling guilty is counterproductive.

You can get back into ketosis quickly with a little trick called "fat-fasting," and you can use it during your feeding window. It is a great way to get back on track, with less hunger or cravings. A fat fast is a high-fat, low-calorie diet used on the IF:45 plan only for one day.

During this time, I recommend that 80 to 90 percent of what you eat comes from fat. Though not technically a fast, this approach mimics the biological effects of abstaining from food by putting your body in ketosis.

Foods you can eat include:

- High-fat meats and fish: bacon, sardines, and salmon
- Eggs: whole eggs and egg yolks
- Oils: coconut oil, MCT oil, olive oil, and avocado oil
- High-fat fruits: avocados and olives
- Non-starchy vegetables like kale, spinach, and zucchini that have been cooked in fat
- Nuts and nut butters
- High-fat, nondairy products: full-fat coconut milk and coconut cream
- Beverages: water, tea, and coffee

Build your meals to include these foods during your feeding window. Stay on this "fast" for no more than one day.

Day 18: Spice it up

Perking up your foods with certain spices during your feeding window can help you on the IF:45 plan. Cinnamon, for example, has been shown to slow gastric emptying, suppress hunger, and lower blood-sugar levels. Add some to your tea or coffee.

Ginger is another spice you can add to tea and coffee. Like cinnamon, it also has blood-sugar regulation benefits.

Nutmeg is a spice you can add to any smoothie, or even tea. Sipping on some nutmeg tea prior to bedtime can help calm you down for a good night's sleep.

Curcumin, an ingredient in the spice turmeric, is known to help boost autophagy. It can also aid weight loss by reducing insulin. Add it to soups, stews, and vegetables.

Salt your foods, too, if you get light-headed or develop headaches while fasting—you may not be getting enough salt. Add some to your food every day.

Day 19: Explore going dairy-free (if you haven't already)

Dairy foods are problematic for many women because they can trigger a number of problems ranging from digestive troubles to weight gain. Why is dairy often a problem? For several reasons. Dairy:

- Can raise insulin
- Is inflammatory (and can cause symptoms like belly bloat)
- Can expose you to synthetic versions of recombinant bovine growth hormone (rBGH) and antibiotics that are given to cows
- Raises IGF-1, a growth factor that in normal amounts possesses certain antiaging benefits but at high levels has been associated with an increased risk for developing some types of cancer and even decreased life span

Dairy can also be addictive because it contains morphine-like compounds. When you digest it, a milk protein called casein is broken down into casomorphin (a morphine-like protein) that crosses the blood-brain barrier and promotes the release of dopamine. Dopamine is that reward/ pleasure chemical in our body that encourages cravings. This is why researchers have referred to dairy products as "dairy crack."

For many years, my dairy consumption was pretty minimal—with the exception of some raw dairy and occasional ice cream. But after I removed all dairy, I dropped that elusive last five-plus pounds of perimenopause weight I had been wanting to lose for several years.

The first few weeks were tough, but I can honestly say, now that I don't consume it, it makes my life so much easier. I will occasionally use high-quality grass-fed butter and ghee, but after three years of being dairy-free, I don't miss it at all. Nut milks are a delicious, much healthier alternative.

Besides dairy, other commonly found inflammatory foods include gluten, processed sugars, grains, and alcohol. They can cause rashes, skin changes, joint pain, headaches, fatigue, difficulty sleeping, bloating, changes in respiration, and digestive issues. If you suspect that foods on this list make you feel uncomfortable, I suggest that you remove them and see what happens. Do what works for you.

Day 20: Get better slumber

The more time you spend sleeping, the more you chip away at your fasting window. Adequate sleep also helps you resist cravings and suppress your hunger hormones.

But if you're still struggling with sleep, here are some additional measures you can add today:

- Supplement with bioidentical GABA (gamma-aminobutyric acid), an amino acid in the brain that serves as a major inhibitory neurotransmitter in the central nervous system. It is also a critical calming agent for the body and helps combat stress and anxiety. Take 200 milligrams of GABA in the evening right before ending your feeding window.
- CBD oil. It is a good sleep promoter because it has a naturally calming effect on the brain and body. This is something to try if your brain just can't shut down properly. It also brings down inflammation.

Other natural sleep supplements to try are:

- L-theanine or an adaptogenic herb such as rhodiola
- A serving of a healthy starchy carbohydrate added to your evening meal
- 1 teaspoon of MCT oil to see if it helps with sleep. My clients tell me this strategy really helps with sleep quality.

Take a break from fasting until you're sleeping better or reduce your fasting window. Make sure you're following the proper recommendations for fasting when cycling. Follow my sleep recommendations on page 140.

How to Select a CBD Oil

Chances are you've found that it's confusing to choose a CBD oil, because there are so many choices on the market. Let me help clear up the confusion. CBD oil is available as CBD isolate, full-spectrum CBD, or broad-spectrum CBD.

CBD isolate is the purest form of CBD, isolated from the other compounds of the hemp plant. CBD isolate should have no THC, one of the active ingredients in the cannabis plant, from which the oil is extracted.

Full-spectrum CBD contains all the naturally available compounds of the cannabis plant, including THC. In a hemp-derived full-spectrum product, the THC content is no more than 0.3 percent of the dry weight. THC levels rise when the flowers are extracted into oil.

Broad-spectrum CBD has all of the naturally occurring compounds except the THC, or it contains very little. Broad-spectrum CBD oil is typically high-quality.

So, which should you choose? Some people prefer full-spectrum because they want all of the cannabis plant's benefits—with all of the cannabinoids and other compounds working in synergy. Others choose broad-spectrum because they want all of the flavonoids and other beneficial plant compounds but no THC. Some people prefer CBD isolate because it's tasteless and odorless, and they don't want any other compounds included.

You might want to experiment with each choice to see which one you like best. Some products are especially formulated for help with sleep and insomnia.

Day 21: Enjoy some chocolate today

As long as it's dark—at least 70 percent cacao or above, chocolate is your healthiest treat on the IF:45 plan. Dark chocolate is:

- Packed with minerals, including iron, magnesium, manganese, potassium, and zinc
- Full of healthy fatty acids
- So rich in antioxidants that a study in the *Chemistry Central Journal* dubbed cacao a "super fruit"
- Stimulates autophagy in the liver cells and in the heart, thanks to phenolic compounds in cacao

Add more cacao to your diet by reaching for a square of dark chocolate. My favorite brand is Hu.

Day 22: Break plateaus

Sometimes, despite your best efforts, you hit a standstill with your weight loss, otherwise known as weight-loss resistance. If you're at that point, here are six ways to power through a plateau.

STOP OVEREXERCISING. If you begin exercising and doing intense cardio multiple days a week—and performing all this on days you've had little sleep and high stress, it is quite possible that your body will go into fat-storing mode, the literal opposite of what you desire! Overexercising overtaxes your hormones, generating too much cortisol (which impacts insulin and blood-sugar control), and sets off a ripple effect of unwanted outcomes, such as weight gain. Be kinder to your body and it will respond accordingly.

Please incorporate deliberate daily activity, but scale back on the intensity. You can resume harder workouts after you've fueled your body properly the day before and you've gotten a good night's sleep. Stick to walking, yoga, Pilates, and strength training rather than chronic cardio. These choices will lower your stress response.

STOP UNDEREATING. Calorie restriction seems to be the logical route toward weight loss, but you can take it too far. When I speak with women and hear about what they are actually eating, I know many are down to 800 to 1,000 calories a day in an attempt to get lean. When you do this, your body thinks it's starving, and to rebel, it will hold on to fat stores.

You must take in a sufficient amount of macros each day. Consume protein and healthy fat with every meal and become very conscientious about carbs. This is a recipe for losing body fat, maintaining a healthy weight, and enhancing longevity.

WORK ON SLEEP. We need seven to nine hours of high-quality sleep, every single night. Peak growth hormone is secreted at night. It helps your body heal and develop lean muscle. Its secretion isn't going to happen unless you get into a deep sleep. If you are waking up between 2:00 and 4:00 a.m., you aren't getting into the deep sleep required for weight loss. Waking up like this indicates poor blood-sugar control, hormone dysregulation, cravings, and appetite issues.

MANAGE STRESS. Too much cortisol can lead to retention of fat tissue. You must prioritize an action plan to handle stress. Whether that be mindfulness, meditation, journaling, or therapy, it must become a part of your daily routine or you will not reduce the cortisol output.

SHORTEN YOUR FEEDING WINDOW. Everyone's metabolism is bio-individual, and it can take different women different lengths of time to reach their goals. To change things up, try working up to a 17:7 or 18:6 model. These help kick-start weight loss.

WAIT IT OUT. Sometimes stubborn fat is just that—stubborn. Your weight may be in limbo for weeks and then, for no apparent reason, start dropping again. Just be patient, give yourself grace, keep doing what you've been doing, and don't give up.

Day 23: Challenge yourself with a protein fast

Changing things up with your fasts is extremely important. Variety is key! Just by adding intermittent fasting into your daily routine, you're already allowing your body to rid itself of toxins and excess hormones.

Now let's supercharge this a bit with a "protein fast." This involves lowering your protein intake slightly and allows your body to use other methods for energy and to perform at its peak. Protein fasts help you reach autophagy and assist with fat loss.

So do a protein fast today. Limit your protein intake to 15 to 25 grams or less for the day (this includes all protein sources, including vegetables). On this day, enjoy a higher fat and moderate-carb meal plan.

Day 24: Troubleshoot fatigue

With intermittent fasting, you should seldom feel fatigued. But because we're all different, you might feel tired on some days. This can be common, so don't let it dissuade you from sticking to your new lifestyle. Some troubleshooting tips to combat fatigue:

- Stay hydrated and don't leave out the electrolytes (see chapter 7)
- Adjust your macros to allow a little more fat
- Get seven to nine hours of sleep every night
- Take a short break from fasting to see how you feel
- Talk to your health care provider if your fatigue does not resolve

Consider where you are in your menstrual cycle; again, no fasting five to seven days preceding your cycle.

Day 25: Engage in mindful movement

Today, make time to do "mindful movements" such as yoga, a nature walk, Pilates, a swim, stretching, or outdoor play. Focus your attention solely on how your body feels when you're moving. This helps you let go of worry and stress and cultivates peace, especially if you feel like everything is out of control. Seek what you do have control over—how you move, breathe, and feel during the activity.

Not every second of exercise has to be high intensity. Additionally, if you've found your normal workouts to be challenging to do while fasted, this might be a good shift to make.

Day 26: Introduce adaptogens into your feeding window

Adaptogens are herbs that help your body naturally combat stress. Stress comes in many forms and we want to naturally support our hormones so they can do their job optimally. These herbs "adapt" to your body and help support its needs.

Besides rhodiola rosea and ashwagandha, I like maca, schisandra, and reishi mushrooms. These are effective to add when you are in your feeding window, particularly maca. Maca is one of my favorites.

Maca is actually a tuber, similar to a turnip, that is in the brassica family with Brussels sprouts, cauliflower, and broccoli. It is indigenous to Peru and is sometimes referred to as Peruvian ginseng. Maca is considered to be a true super food because of all of its amazing properties!

Maca is helpful on the IF:45 plan because it helps balance hormones in women. It supports the hypothalamus-pituitary-adrenal axis (HPA), which is involved in orchestrating communication between our thyroid, ovaries, and adrenals. These organs need special attention as women age and go through perimenopause and menopause.

Besides being an adaptogenic herb, maca can help regulate blood sugar. It also can improve energy and libido levels. It is rich in vitamins and minerals like magnesium, zinc, potassium, and iron and full of plant sterols and fatty acids. All of these contribute to energy regulation, satiety, and better sleep.

Before supplementing with maca or adding in lots of supplements, it is reasonable to have a DUTCH test, a special dried urine and saliva test. To find a provider that uses this test, go to www.dutchtest.com. This is one of my favorite tests to incorporate with my mature clients. It provides insights into how we metabolize sex hormones, cortisol, DHEA, melatonin, and many others. It can help fill conceptual gaps by providing a full clinical picture on how best to address lifestyle, nutritional issues, and fasting.

Day 27: Make good use of your extra time

You probably haven't thought much about it, but a lot of your day used to revolve around eating, especially during the days of three meals and snacks daily. Many of us have structured our days around mealtimes.

So now, with intermittent fasting, you don't have to do all that because you're not eating much of the time. That break in your routine might feel jarring at first, with lots of idle time that you don't know how to fill.

In reality, you have more time now! So fill it with non-food activities that you couldn't fit in before: daily physical activity, meditation, self-care activities (massages, facials, and so forth), quality time with friends or family, projects you've put on hold, and so forth.

Day 28: Prepare bone broth

Bone broth (or vegetable broth) has a special place in my IF:45 plan, because it has a powerful effect on your microbiome, which is essential to digestive and immune health. It is high in minerals and collagen, plus helps manage hunger. The longer you cook it (twelve to twenty-four hours), the more collagen it yields. Make some today and store it in your fridge. You can also freeze it for the future.

If you're time-crunched, you can purchase premade bone broth. Make sure it's organic and non-GMO. A good brand is Kettle Fire, which makes many different flavors.

Day 29: Do a twenty-four-hour fast

This involves going without food for twenty-four hours. I implement this strategy once a month. To be successful, ensure that you consume proper calories the day before from protein, healthy fats, and carbs. Staying well hydrated is also key. I always look forward to these, especially when I feel like my body needs a "reset" after vacation, parties, and so forth.

Personally, it's easiest for me to fast from dinner one day until dinner the next, but the timing is completely up to you. But again, don't push a longer fast if you are not ready to do so!

Day 30: Add some natural sugars to your meals

Hopefully by this point, you've eliminated processed sugars. Sugar is endemic in processed foods, and evidence shows that it can be highly addictive and inflammatory. It hinders your body's ability to detoxify itself by harming key detoxifying organs like the liver. It is also a culprit in insulin resistance, type 2 diabetes, obesity, heart disease, and possibly Alzheimer's disease because of its inflammatory properties.

If that isn't enough, sugar accelerates the aging process by increasing a process called glycation, in which sugar molecules link with protein molecules and cause wrinkling and the degradation of collagen and elastin in the skin.

The good news is that you can enjoy some sugar—but only the natural kind found in fruits. Here is a list of fruits lower in sugar. Be sure to watch your portions and balance these with a little protein or healthy fat. However, if you are insulin resistant and your body is not properly burning carbohydrates (metabolic inflexibility), you should probably avoid sugar or keep your portions exceedingly small.

- Stone fruits
- Berries
- Apples
- Citrus fruits

Day 31: Adopt the "good, better, best" mindset

I've always believed in progress, not perfection, and this is where the "good, better, best" mindset comes in. In a perfect world, I exercise every day, I prepare healthy meals for my family, I establish the perfect fasting and feeding windows, and I get all my work done for the day.

You know as well as I do that things pop up . . . the Internet goes down, social events intervene, something comes up with the kids, or there's no time to prep meals. This is when I've learned to adopt the "good, better, best" mindset to help me get through my plan while still sticking to my goals.

Here's how this works:

Best is the perfect day. You can stick to your schedule of fasting, working out, preparing and eating a healthy meal, meeting your work and family obligations, and going to bed on time. You even have time for relaxation.

Better is a day when things get a little hectic. You might have to skip your workout, order a healthy take-out meal, or table some commitments for another day. It's not a "best" day. But you did your best and are still on track.

Good is when things go haywire. Maybe you were able to stick to only one thing—like a healthy meal plan—or you got in fifteen minutes of working out rather than an hour. Pat yourself on the back. It is okay because you still accomplished something. Never think you messed up! You still have forward momentum.

There may be days you DO give up or ALL your healthy habits go out the window for some reason or another. Regardless, you have not stopped making forward progress forever. There is always a new day ahead!

This mindset works for my clients and for the participants in my master classes. Said Terry: "I've been intermittent fasting for a year, but it wasn't until I adopted the good, better, best approach that I became consistent. As a result, I got the results I wanted—which was primarily in long-term brain health. I feel mentally sharper and my mood and attitude toward life is more positive than it has ever been."

The upside of this mindset is that it gets you out of perfection mode, which can be paralyzing. It also liberates you from an "all or nothing" mentality. A lot of people feel that if they don't give something 100 percent all the time, they've failed, so they give up on the entire plan. There is no strict set of rules on IF:45, only best, better, good options you can weigh every day. Sure, "best" is ideal, but better is better than you've done in the past, and good is still making progress. The only option that isn't acceptable is giving up!

Day 32: Protect and detox your skin

While you're working on your body on the IF:45 plan, let's talk about protecting it from environmental toxins and xenoestrogens by changing up your skin care routine.

Our skin is an organ—the largest organ, in fact. And because our skin is porous, it absorbs any and everything we put on it: creams, lotions, perfumes, deodorants, shampoos, conditioners, nail polish, and more, and all the chemicals and toxins these products contain.

A significant consequence of built-up toxin exposure from skin care products is hormonal imbalance, because many products contain xenoestrogens, which act like or affect estrogen inside the body. There are thousands of such chemicals, and their multitude is mind-boggling.

That being so, start hunting for skin care products in the same way that you choose foods for a healthy diet: look for natural ingredients, without any harsh chemicals or anything artificial!

So today, commit to changing your skincare routine to protect your body from toxins and hormone disruptors. Some strategies:

- Stick to an anti-inflammatory diet (no gluten. no grains, no dairy, and limited processed sugars) to fight toxins
- Prioritize quality sleep and use a Slip eye mask (silk) with a silk pillowcase
- Try coconut oil–based products for skin and hair care to cleanse, moisturize, and remove makeup
- Use apple cider vinegar to cleanse the skin of harmful bacteria
- Make homemade facial scrubs with sea salt for exfoliation
- Have a consistent skin care regimen—morning and evening. Your skin likes routine! Mine involves a facial wash, eye cream, moisturizer, vitamin serums, and biweekly exfoliation—all with products free of toxins and harsh chemicals. See my Best Practices, in the Appendix, for a list of recommended products.

Days 33–34: Tackle leptin resistance

This is an important health issue, so let's work on it over a two-day period. Quite often leptin resistance and insulin resistance go hand in hand. Similar to insulin resistance, over time your body can produce too much leptin and you become desensitized to it. Here are some signs that you may be leptin resistant:

- Belly fat
- High blood glucose levels

- High reverse T3 (This is an inactive form of the thyroid hormone T3. A high reverse T3 may indicate a low metabolism, which leads to weight gain. Symptoms of a high reverse T3 include fatigue, depression, low blood pressure, and a slower-than-normal pulse rate.)
- Low energy
- Not feeling satiated after meals
- Not losing weight; hitting plateaus
- Sweet cravings

Fortunately, there are many tools you can use to help support leptin sensitivity, including intermittent fasting. For example:

- Add electrolytes to your water, including magnesium (see chapter 7)
- Aim for thirty minutes a day of exercise or movement
- Avoid toxins in food and products you use
- Don't snack and don't eat after dinner
- Eat organic, grass-fed, and non-GMO foods
- Eliminate all processed sugar
- Enjoy healthy fats
- Focus on gut health and strategies for proper elimination
- Emphasize protein at meals
- Stay low-carb
- Incorporate anti-inflammatory foods into your diet
- Reduce stress
- Aim for seven to nine hours of uninterrupted sleep each night
- Get daily sun exposure in order to increase vitamin D levels, which will help with inflammation

Day 35: Evaluate non-scale victories

I think it's fine to weigh yourself on the scale periodically—but not obsessively. Your scale gives you a number—a snapshot of your weight at a given moment on a given day. But the journey to a healthier life can't be reduced to a snapshot so easily. I prefer that you look at non-scale victories—health improvements that result from lifestyle changes. They are a much better measure of your success.

So for today, evaluate your non-scale victories by asking yourself a series of questions:

Do my clothes fit better than they used to?
Do I feel more energized to do things like playing with my children or pets, working in my garden, or enjoying a hike in nature?
Has my sleep improved?
Does my mind feel sharper and more focused?
Does my skin look clearer?
Do I have less pain?
Is my mood brighter?
Are my cravings disappearing?
Have my medical markers (blood pressure, blood sugar, lipids, and so forth) improved?

When you can answer most of these questions affirmatively, this can boost your resolve and reassure you that your lifestyle changes have improved your health.

Day 36: Tap into the spirituality of fasting

Intermittent fasting is immensely powerful in the mental and spiritual realm. Studies have shown that intermittent fasters report unusual mental clarity during their fasting windows. Not eating helps the brain clean out toxic debris and may even help prevent dementia as you get older.

As I've mentioned, fasting is also anti-inflammatory, which directly affects brain functioning, too. And of course, intermittent fasting prompts growth in the mitochondria, resulting in sharper cognitive function—and may even explain why spiritual fasters report such amazing insights and visions.

So today, as you withdraw from the daily demands of feeding your body, focus on what's left—bigger-picture items such as what direction you want your life to take or manifesting the achievement of your goals.

Day 37: Cultivate gratitude

Gratitude is defined as the quality of being grateful or the readiness to show appreciation for and to return kindness. The word "readiness" really is the key because you can sail through life professing being grateful, without fully appreciating what that really represents in its true whole form.

As Ralph Waldo Emerson put it: "Cultivate the habit of being grateful for every good thing that comes to you, and to give thanks continuously. And because all things have contributed to your advancement, you should include all things in your gratitude."

So, how can you go about creating this ritual and habit? Some suggestions:

- Practice gratitude journaling. You may think you don't have time to journal, but you actually do. Simply commit to writing down three things you are grateful for each day. They can be mundane—like sunshine instead of rain or not missing the bus—but they are powerful!
- Follow the advice of Dutch philosopher Rabbi Baruch Spinoza. He believed you should ask yourself three questions each day: (1) Who or what inspired me today? (2) What brought me happiness today? (3) What brought me comfort and deep peace today?
- Write your answers in your journal and reflect upon them.

- After fasting and entering your feeding window, approach the act of filling your stomach with pure gratitude for the gift of the food itself and how it is nourishing your body.
- Keep yourself in a positive mindset. Today, finish this sentence:
  - I am proud of myself for _____.

To view the 5 references cited in this chapter, please visit cynthiathurlow.com/references.

Chapter 11

. . . .

Phase 3: Modification—
Days 38 to 45

Congratulations! You have entered the final week of the IF:45 plan—the Modification Phase. Here, we take intermittent fasting to a new level, with some advanced variations now that you've mastered the basics. For example, I'll have you try some extended fasting, in which you go for a day without eating. Evidence keeps accumulating that not only does an extended fast supercharge the benefits of intermittent fasting—like faster weight loss—it also results in more profound changes to health markers like better blood-sugar control and growth-hormone surges.

And, according to studies, extended fasting reduces ghrelin (the appetite-boosting hormone), so you may actually become less hungry on a longer fast. Some people even report a rush of feel-good endorphins with extended fasting. This is probably why longer fasts have such a rich spiritual and religious history.

Results like these are borne out by other research. One fairly recent study, published in *PLOS ONE*, followed more than fourteen hundred people over one year. They participated in a program consisting of fasting periods of between four and twenty-one days (in this study, "fasting" allowed a daily calorie intake of 200 to 250 calories). Among all fasting lengths, the study found significant reductions in weight, waistline circumference, and blood pressure, as well as improvements in blood lipids (cholesterol and triglycerides) and blood-sugar regulation. Among the 404 people who had preexisting health complaints, 84 percent reported improvements.

Perhaps the most striking of all is that 93 percent of the participants said they felt an increase in physical and emotional well-being and had an absence of hunger. Although the participants were taking in some calories, extended fasts are not for everyone. The point of this study is really to underline the positive health benefits of fasting. The researchers concluded that "periodic fasting from four to 21 days is safe and well-tolerated."

Science aside, participants in my master classes have been able to easily do extended fasting at times. Taylor is a good example. By the time she was well into the Modification Phase, she told me, "I can do extended fasts without any issues, and one reason is that I have changed physically, emotionally, and mentally—all for the better." Among those changes, Taylor said she lost 80 percent of her love handles, along with eight pounds, and she no longer feels fatigued—which had been a huge problem for her in the past.

Results you can expect from the Modification Phase:

- More fat loss
- Boosted autophagy
- Fewer cravings
- More insulin sensitivity
- Better balanced hormones
- Reduced inflammation
- More mental clarity

Continue to follow my menu plans on pages 221–222, adjusting where needed.

Day 38: Vary your fasting days

Our bodies actually get bored with the same routine, just like we do. They need something different from time to time. It keeps them guessing—and responding better to fasting. Starting today and for the next week, I want you to schedule the following:

- five regular intermittent fasting days
- one extended fast (aim for twenty-four hours or longer)
- one feast day

Your feast day is a time when you lengthen your feeding window and consume more food. Do not confuse this with a binge day and eating everything in your kitchen. Instead, have three meals that day instead of your regular two or one (depending on your regular fasting schedule) over a twelve-hour feeding window. Enjoy some starchy carbs (sweet potato, beans, lentils, and so forth) with your meals, particularly if you strength train (see Day 39). Feast days remind your body that it's not starving.

Day 39: Extend safely

One important element of longer fasts is that they require a little more oversight. You can safely plan a fast that goes beyond twenty-four hours (as recommended above). Some people go for even longer fasts, such as thirty, thirty-six, or even forty-two hours. With any extended fast, it is a good idea to consult your health care practitioner, especially if you are on medication for diabetes, high blood pressure, or another chronic condition.

Then watch for signs. If you feel sick, weak, or faint, stop fasting and see your doctor. Try to stay busy and keep a normal schedule. Hydrate often with water and electrolytes, as well as with coffee or tea—both of which help suppress hunger and boost fat-burning.

Day 40: Adjust your macros on more intense exercise days

If you have been successful with fat loss on IF:45, you may decide it's time to focus on muscle gain instead, with higher-intensity workouts. Or if you're constantly feeling drained in energy on exercise days, you may need to make a few dietary changes, too. Situations like these call for an entirely new macro setup.

Experts typically recommend the following macro breakdown when you are focused on muscle-building:

Carbohydrates: 40 to 50 percent of total daily calories
Protein: 30 to 40 percent of total daily calories
Fat: 20 to 30 percent of total daily calories

Remember that we are all unique and bio-individual. What works great for one woman may not necessarily work best for you. It's all about figuring out your own system and how you are responding to various macros.

Here are some suggestions on how to rework your macros and shift them around a bit.

Carbohydrates

If you're focused on building lean muscle and working out harder to do it, add more carbs back to your day. Carbs help keep you in an anabolic state, building muscle as quickly as possible, especially if you strength train. As a side note, I highly recommend strength training for women. Strength training helps build skeletal muscle, which we lose with age. Strength training can help burn calories long after we have finished our sessions. It also helps build stronger bones and create insulin sensitivity, among other benefits.

Strength training is an anaerobic activity, meaning that its energy production pathway runs on glucose and carbohydrates. It can't use fats or ketones. So if you strength train several days a week, your body requires a few more carbohydrates than usual—but just enough to properly fuel and recover from your workouts, without any excess being stored as body fat, or causing insulin problems. So—how do you get there? I suggest adding in a serving a day of quality carbohydrates such as ⅓ cup sweet potato or a small sweet potato, ⅓ cup of winter squash, or ⅓ cup of beans or lentil. See how your energy levels are during your workouts. If your energy feels low, you can add an additional serving of carbohydrates to your diet. Everyone is different due to bio-individuality. Listen to your body.

Also, if you have good insulin sensitivity, or you strength train at a very high intensity, you can adjust your carbs upward on workout days. If you have poor insulin sensitivity, and work out on the lower end of training intensity or are working on losing fat, stick to the lower range on training days.

When adjusting your carb intake, make the right choices. In addition to non-starchy vegetables (which contain some carbs) and low-sugar fruits, I recommend selecting starches that provide the proper fuel for strength training. The majority of your added starchy carbs should come from root vegetables such as yams and sweet potatoes; winter squashes; and beans and legumes—rather than from grains or gluten-containing carbs—as I noted above.

Protein

With more intense workouts, you need more protein because it is essential for building, repairing, and maintaining body tissues and is involved in metabolism and hormone systems.

On average, a protein intake of 1 gram per pound or more can be beneficial if you are involved in an intense strength training program. Your perfect protein number also depends on your body size as well as the type and length of your workouts. If a healthy weight for your height and stature is 135 pounds, then your goal should be 135 grams of protein daily. That's the equivalent of 6 ounces each of a lean steak, chicken breast, and a salmon fillet.

Fat

As for fat, it is generally recommended that if you strength train several times a week, your fat intake should be 0.4 grams of fat per pound of body weight per day. Using the example of someone who weighs 135 pounds, that person would eat 54 grams of fat daily. That is the equivalent of one avocado and about 2 tablespoons of olive oil.

Day 41: Use brain-boosting nutritional strategies

The research is clear: Intermittent fasting sharpens mental acuity, increases focus and concentration, clears away brain fog, and wards off the chances of neurodegenerative diseases such as Alzheimer's. In fact, even if you have no interest in losing weight or improving health markers, the positive benefits of fasting on the brain alone are amazing.

In addition to improved cognitive functioning, fasting can reduce the effects of aging on your brain. It also strengthens stress resistance and reduces inflammation. Fasting also increases brain-derived neurotrophic factors (BDNF). The longer the fast, the more BDNF, which helps prevent brain degenerative diseases.

It is remarkable that just by delaying eating your food, not only are you giving your gut digestive rest, but you are also helping your mind clear out all the junk as well. You may notice that you have more energy or your usual afternoon slump has disappeared. You should feel more focused and more driven to reach your goals and accomplish things you set out to do.

During your eating window, you can support your brain's newfound fitness by feeding it with brain-boosting foods. Today, consider building your meal plans around some of these key foods:

- Omega-3 fatty acid–rich foods like salmon and other fatty fish and walnuts. Omega-3 fatty acids improve blood circulation and enhance the function of neurotransmitters, which help your brain process and think.

- Foods high in magnesium, such as chickpeas. They help with message transmission in your brain.
- Blueberries, which are associated with quicker learning, better thinking, and greater memory retention.
- Choline-rich foods, such as broccoli and cauliflower. They can help with the growth of new brain cells, as well as boosting intelligence as you get older.

Day 42 to 44: Take the 30:16 challenge

There is a type of extreme time-restricted fast called the one-meal-a-day (OMAD) plan. I normally don't recommend it because it is one of the most challenging plans to follow and can be a big adjustment. It is also difficult to get all of your nutrients in a single meal.

That said, I have a three-day technique I'd like you to try that still embodies one meal a day: my 30:16 plan. It is an effective advanced strategy that changes up the timing of your meals. You keep your body guessing when its next meal is, as well as reaping the benefits of longer fasts.

Here's how it works.

- Eat your OMAD for dinner Monday evening. Go heavy on lean protein, healthy fats, leafy greens, and other non-starchy vegetables. It is also a good idea to include a serving of a starchy vegetable carbohydrate such as a sweet potato or ½ cup of beans or legumes.
- Fast for sixteen hours following your dinner, and eat lunch Tuesday afternoon. Have a lean protein, healthy fat, and leafy greens or other non-starchy vegetables.
- Following that lunch, fast for thirty hours and eat dinner Wednesday evening. Dinner can be a meal of lean protein, healthy fats, leafy greens, and other non-starchy vegetables, as well as a serving of a starchy vegetable carbohydrate.

Trying this plan several times a month can be highly effective for weight loss, weight maintenance, fat adaptation, insulin sensitivity, and other positive health markers.

Day 45: Celebrate your transformation

An important part of your intermittent fasting journey is to celebrate your transformation—physically, emotionally, and spiritually. You did the work and it's time to reward yourself for it!

The question is: What is the best way to celebrate these milestones? It is definitely not to go out and splurge on a huge pizza. Don't worry: There are still fun and exciting yet healthy ways to celebrate what you've accomplished. Some ideas:

- Schedule a spa day for all-day pampering and self-care.
- Buy some new workout clothes.
- Enjoy an afternoon to yourself doing something you love. Meet a close friend for coffee, visit a local art museum, take a walk or a hike in nature, go shopping for new clothes, or go for a drive in the country to unwind and refocus.
- Attend a new yoga, Zumba, or dance class.
- Treat yourself to a portrait or boudoir photography session.
- Get a massage.
- Try a new haircut or color to go with your new you.

The possibilities for celebration are limited only by your imagination!

To view the 5 references cited in this chapter,
please visit cynthiathurlow.com/references.

Chapter 12

Maintain Your Intermittent Fasting Lifestyle

A comment that has echoed throughout my master classes is this one, expressed by Elaine, a fifty-year-old participant who had spent most of her adult life on the diet merry-go-round, losing and regaining weight almost every year: "I'm sticking with intermittent fasting. It's completely normal for me now. I cannot imagine going back to what I used to do and how I used to eat. Intermittent fasting is my lifestyle now, and I feel wonderful."

You may have started IF:45 to lose weight but, like Elaine, by now you have discovered many other benefits and want to maintain those benefits. Remember that research has shown that intermittent fasting can help you lose weight and keep it off, but it does more than that, including:

- Greater energy
- Fewer cravings
- Less brain fog
- Greater metabolic health
- Lower blood pressure
- Improved blood-sugar control
- Insulin sensitivity
- Hormonal balance
- Antiaging and increased longevity

In other words, intermittent fasting not only results in weight loss. It transforms health!

If you've experienced any of these benefits, you're probably hooked on intermittent fasting by now. That's good, because it is more than a short-term plan to access some benefits; it's a lifestyle you can sustain for the rest of your life. And I hope you're thinking that it is one of the best decisions you've ever made—and that you definitely want to continue it.

After all, intermittent fasting is so natural! Our bodies are attuned to fasting because it's how our ancestors evolved, and our metabolisms work better when operating on a fasted/fed schedule. Many of our modern health problems can be directly linked to eating too much and too often. Fasting solves all this by limiting the window during which we can eat—so it's something you want to maintain. This may be the end of the forty-five-day intermittent fast, but it is the beginning of a whole new lifestyle for you.

So—let's talk about the strategies you can now incorporate for long-term success throughout your lifetime.

Create Your Plan for the Future

From here on out, intermittent fasting as a lifestyle may mean a different pattern for you. Perhaps you can fast using 16:8 on weekdays, with a three-meal-a-day plan on Saturday and Sunday. Or maybe you do some longer, more intensive fasts during the week. For example:

20:4
For a more intense fast, you can try 20:4, in which you do a twenty-hour fast and a four-hour window in which to eat.

24-Hour Fast
During a twenty-four-hour fast, you'll fast for a full day. Many people who fast for twenty-four hours will only do this once or twice a week. On non-fasting days, they eat as usual. Some people continue on with this way of

eating for the long term, however, and practice the one-meal-a-day (OMAD) pattern, which is also extremely beneficial to weight control and overall health, as long as you take in enough nutrients.

36-Hour Fast

Here, you would eat dinner at 7:00 p.m. on day 1, skip all meals on day 2, and eat breakfast at 7:00 a.m. on day 3.

42-Hour Fast

On this fast, follow the pattern above, but extend your fast on day 3 until 1:00 p.m.

Clearly, there are many ways to incorporate intermittent fasting into your lifestyle. You may need to experiment for a while to work out what suits you best. Very important: If you undertake a longer fast, please consult your health care provider.

Stop Your Fasting Plan When Necessary

I get a lot of questions about what to do when someone has a vacation or business travel coming up. Unlike most "diets," intermittent fasting (which is not a diet!) is so flexible that you can do it while traveling—if you want to—and not miss a beat, or not do it and ease back into it after your trip.

I know this from personal experience. I've had an increase in travel in the last year, and my travel has been largely work-related. I've enjoyed the experience immensely. Travel is a major part of my soul because I love experiencing new people and new places. Amazingly, I've found that my eating style—which is strictly gluten-free, grain-free, and dairy-free, with a high priority on protein consumption—is pretty easy to follow. And so is intermittent fasting.

When traveling, I maintain a 16:8 fasting window, the same pattern I do at home. It's the easiest to follow, especially on long airplane flights.

I usually break my fast with an egg dish. Just about everywhere I go, I can find an omelet or egg option. I love eggs. They are the perfect balance of protein and fat, and gentle on my digestive system. I take every opportunity for extra protein. If a restaurant serves steak or chicken, I'm ordering it. I try to load up on protein when I can so I can enjoy myself when carbs are the only option, which is often the case in other countries. I also prioritize other proteins when I'm dining out. And of course, I load up on veggies and salads—which are easy to find on menus.

If you decide to do intermittent fasting while on a trip, it's okay to shift or shorten your feeding window to make your vacation more fun or convenient.

Nor do you even need to fast. You're probably not on vacation alone. You're usually with friends or your family, and it isn't fun to be fasting when everyone else wants to eat meals together. Enjoying your vacation is just as important as everything else.

So give yourself permission to take a vacation from fasting. Eat breakfast with your family and friends. Enjoy other meals. Don't miss out on vacation fun. If you want to take a vacation from fasting, that's totally fine.

Extra meals here and there aren't going to make a difference, I promise you. My best advice for this isn't exactly big news: Don't stress about it. Stress will throw your hormones out of balance and interfere with your sleep—both of which do damage to your system. Get back on your feeding/fasting schedule once you get home.

If you're worried about weight gain or slowing your metabolism, try to get as much walking and activity as you can by enjoying the sights and the outdoors.

If you're traveling for a month, or two months, or some other extended amount of time, you might need to be a little more disciplined. But intermittent fasting, especially 16:8, is so easy and painless that it doesn't feel like discipline.

Once you're back from your trip, you might find it difficult to adjust to your feeding/fasting strategy after a week or two of taking it easy.

The best way to reacclimate is to take it slowly. You might have to begin with a shorter fasting window and ease back into the 16:8 pattern. Resume your normal, healthy meals during your feeding window. Get back into your workout routine. Your body will quickly get back into the swing of things.

Make the Right Food Choices for Your Bio-individuality

During your feeding window, eat combinations of healthy foods that I've talked about throughout this book: lean proteins, non-starchy vegetables, healthy fats, and starchy carbohydrates—adjusted according to your macronutrient and cycling needs.

Also, I believe it is essential to listen to your body in terms of how your food choices make you feel. For example, if you feel fatigued after having rice or grains, try eating more non-starchy vegetables instead. See if you feel more energized afterward. If so, your body is telling you to stick to veggies and stay away from grains.

Continue to change things up by altering your macros, especially if you're cycling. Our bodies are constantly changing as we get older. Plus, eating the same meals every day increases the odds of developing food intolerances and sensitivities.

The key lesson here is to consistently listen to your body and experiment with different foods for optimal health.

Track Your Weight

Staying at your new lower, healthier weight is challenging. Of the millions of people who lose weight each year, only a small number manage to keep the pounds off. The numbers quoted range from 2 percent to 20 percent.

It can be all too easy to get a little complacent and regain weight without really noticing unless you monitor it. If you find that you're putting weight back on, go back to the Induction Phase, in which you lowered your carb intake. Stick with lower carbs and intermittent fasting until you've lost that extra weight.

Decide on an acceptable weight range beyond which you need to take action—a five-pound ceiling, for example. Once you exceed five pounds, you want to get back on track with intermittent fasting, lower carbs, and consistent exercise. In fact, intermittent fasting has been shown in research to be one of the best ways to maintain a desirable weight.

So get right back on your program quickly if your weight strays out of your acceptable target. The longer you let it go, the harder it may be to lose.

Pump Up Your Results with Variations in Daily Exercise

Exercise is a cornerstone of any healthy lifestyle. From our circulatory and respiratory systems to our muscles and joints, our bodies were made to move with beautiful fluidity. When we stop moving, either due to a sedentary lifestyle or for health reasons, our bodies can suffer. We develop stiff joints, excess weight, and poor overall health.

Moving keeps us healthy, and it keeps us happy. Even if you have some limitations for health or ability reasons, exercise is essential for good health. As I've pointed out, exercise works exceptionally well with intermittent fasting. There is evidence that exercising in a fasted state can boost insulin sensitivity and help keep your blood-sugar levels stable, plus help you burn fat faster.

Working out improves mitochondrial function, which makes you more efficient at burning energy. Working out with low glycogen/carb storage specifically trains your mitochondria to burn more fat.

Keep up your daily exercise, with intense workouts like strength training or HIIT two to four times a week. The rest of the week, incorporate more gentle and restorative forms of exercise. Some suggestions:

Walking
You don't have to do a ten-mile run to get a good cardio workout. Walking at a fast pace (aka power walking) can be just as beneficial to your heart as a good run, but with much less physical impact on your body. Walking is easier on your joints. Studies are showing that people who walk while listening to lighthearted podcasts can reduce their cortisol outputs at great rates. Try walking at a fast pace—fast enough to where you can't talk without being out of breath—while pumping your arms. Do this for at least thirty minutes, and you've got a solid cardio routine.

Swimming
Swimming is the ultimate low-impact exercise that is gentle on the joints. It is a common physical therapy modality for many. Swimming provides

an aerobic workout that works every muscle in your body . . . this is why a "swimmer's body" is an enviable physique! There is just something so healing about the water. We reach another level when we submerge ourselves in water and let the stress of our lives slide away. Whether you calmly glide through the water or concentrate on faster-paced strokes, your body will benefit from swimming.

Tai Chi

Tai Chi is an ancient Chinese martial arts tradition that is now practiced as a form of exercise involving a series of movements accompanied by deep breathing. Often called meditation in motion, Tai Chi is a well-known stress reducer. The health benefits of this weight-bearing exercise are numerous and include improving balance and flexibility, preventing falls, and acting as a mood booster. Tai Chi is wonderful for people of all ages and fitness levels. Check with your local Parks & Rec department to see if they offer any group meetups. You could make a few new friends and gain health benefits.

Yoga

Yoga is my personal favorite! Yoga is now so mainstream that you can learn more and start a practice right this very second. Doing even a little yoga every day can make a huge impact in your overall health. There is Vinyasa Flow, Hatha Yoga, Hot Yoga, but I would suggest starting with Yin Yoga. This is a gentle, basic style of yoga that focuses on individual poses and deep focus on the breath. Many local libraries host yoga classes, there are yoga studios nationwide, but most accessible is the Internet. You can find free yoga sessions from expert yogis on YouTube and other search engines. There are free yoga apps for your phone, books, magazines, and more, all dedicated to yoga! Dust off that yoga mat you've got stashed in the back of your closet and get your practice going!

Stretching

You may experience headaches, sore shoulders, sore back, maybe even a stiff jaw that happens when you're particularly stressed. That's because stress makes your muscles tense up and become sore! Stretching is a great way to combat this issue. I try to stretch as much as possible, fitting it in whenever I can. It's easy to do a stretch here and there when you're doing chores or even when you watch TV. Of course, yoga is a great means to a good stretch, but you don't have to achieve a yoga pose when you stretch. Really, it's just any way of gently lengthening a muscle. Do what feels good to you. I particularly like doing some gentle stretches at the end of the day while the family is enjoying TV time and winding down.

As always, listen to your body. If you tune in, your body will tell you how much you can handle and when it's time to add more vigor to your routine.

Monitor Your Metabolic Flexibility

As a reminder, metabolic flexibility is the ability of your body to switch back and forth between fat and carbohydrates for fuel, based on their availability. The more metabolically flexible you are, the less you have to micromanage your macronutrients. You can just eat and, as long as you stick to whole foods, the satiety signaling you receive will be accurate and reliable.

Thus, you want to maintain your metabolic flexibility. To do that, monitor it. This involves paying attention to certain symptoms by periodically asking yourself these questions and hopefully answering in the affirmative:

Are you in a state of mild ketosis each morning? You can gauge this by measuring the ketones in your urine using special test strips available at any pharmacy. Metabolically flexible people will quickly switch to the "fasted" state upon cessation of food overnight—and this will show up as ketosis in the morning.

Can you eat carbohydrates at meals without feeling sleepy afterward?
Can you skip a meal without issue?
Are you snacking less—or not at all?

When you do intermittent fasting now, does it seem easier?

If you achieved your weight loss goal through intermittent fasting, have you been able to maintain that weight loss? (If so, this means that your body is fat-adapted and, therefore, it is easier to keep the weight off.)

Are you able to work out more intensely?

Are your energy levels consistently higher?

Do you feel like your mood has improved—and stabilized?

If you monitor your glucose readings, is your blood sugar staying regulated and stable?

If you answered "yes," to a majority of these questions, congratulations! You are metabolically flexible.

On the other hand, if you are not metabolically flexible, there are actions you can take to regain it.

Make sure you're exercising daily. Regular training—both strength and aerobic—directly counters metabolic inflexibility by addressing the two main offending factors. Exercise increases insulin sensitivity and restores fat-burning. Certain types of training, like HIIT, actually help create new mitochondria. Between improved insulin sensitivity, restored fat-burning, and more (and better) mitochondria, exercise is super-important for regaining metabolic flexibility.

Restore fat adaptation. You can do this with low-carb eating and intermittent fasting throughout the week. Along with exercise, this enhances mitochondrial function, restores fat-burning, and increases insulin sensitivity. Stay with this for about a month. Afterward, you can adjust your carbohydrate level to match your training intensity. Emphasize foods and nutrients that support metabolic flexibility: magnesium, which helps prevent insulin resistance; polyphenols, plant compounds found in dark chocolate and colorful vegetables; and omega-3 fats, which improve mitochondrial function.

Take Advantage of Your Newfound Free Time

Nowadays, your life is a lot simpler. You have more free time to focus on what really matters. No longer will you spend countless hours on meal planning and meal preparation. You've streamlined your days and freed up your nights. There's no more snacking, no more grazing, and less sluggish post-meal periods wondering why you ate so much.

With more time (and money) on your hands, how will you spend it?

Take this newfound freedom and pursue other passions. What has gotten shoved to the back burner before now: advanced education, hobbies, work pursuits, family? Now that you've got extra time in your days, you can spend it on anything you'd like. You might even find some new avenues to explore. The sky's the limit, and IF will open up not just a new world but a whole new universe of opportunities.

To view the 4 references cited in this chapter,
please visit cynthiathurlow.com/references.

Chapter 13

· · · · · · · · · · · · · ·

The IF:45 Meal Plans

To get the most benefits from intermittent fasting, make sure you're eating nutrient-rich foods during your feeding window. Building balanced meals using whole foods—lean proteins, healthy fats, and fiber-rich carbohydrates—will fuel your body, balance your hormones, and build your health during your fast.

This six-week meal plan is organized according to the phases of intermittent fasting: Induction, Optimization, and Modification. The Induction days are all low-carb so that your body can move into ketosis and become more fat-adapted as you fast. With Optimization and Modification, carbohydrates increase most days to a moderate level, but with some low-carb and high-carb days (this is the essence of carb cycling) interspersed in the plan.

If you want to alter your meal setup for even higher carbs during Optimization and Modification, all you have to do is add one small portion of a higher-carb food to one or both of your meals. I've included some examples for you in the chart on page 216. As you begin living the IF lifestyle, small adjustments in your macro intake will offer more and better ways to fuel your fast.

The recipes begin on page 223.

Breakfast Every Day

Black coffee, green tea, or herbal tea

Water with electrolytes (be sure to hydrate throughout the day)

Induction

WEEK 1

Monday

Lunch: 4 pieces Classic Deviled Eggs (page 274), 4 Sausage-Stuffed
Mushrooms (page 292)

Dinner: Skirt Steak with Avocado-Horseradish Cream (page 223),
sautéed green beans

Tuesday

Lunch: Tuna Puttanesca–Stuffed Tomatoes (page 252)

Dinner: Creamy Pesto Chicken-Spinach Casserole
(page 250)

Wednesday

Lunch: 1 Pork-Apple Sausage Patty (page 238), 2 eggs scrambled
with chopped onion and sliced mushrooms

Dinner: Steak Caesar Salad (page 230)

Thursday

Lunch: Creamy Pesto Chicken-Spinach Casserole (page 250)

Dinner: Lamb Shoulder Chops with Olive-Parsley Gremolata
(page 232)

Friday

Lunch: Chilled Cucumber-Avocado Soup with Spicy Shrimp
(page 248)

Dinner: Classic Pulled Pork (page 245), green salad with oil and
vinegar

Saturday

Lunch: Spicy Bison Chili (page 236)

Dinner: Kimchi Shrimp Fried "Rice" (page 247)

Sunday
> Lunch: Fennel, Shallot, and Goat Cheese Frittata (page 270)
> Dinner: Classic Pulled Pork (page 245), green salad with oil and
> vinegar

Healthy Carbs to Cycle in Your Feeding Window

Remember that carb cycling means staggering the amount of carbs you eat over the course of a week. On some days, you eat more carbs, and on others, you eat fewer carbs. Carb cycling gives you the benefits of carbs on some days, and the benefits of eating low-carb on other days—the best of both worlds. For example, the lower-carb days help with weight loss and insulin sensitivity. The higher-carb days assist in replenishing glycogen and supporting muscle growth.

When you eat carbs, make sure they are healthy carbs, not junk food. Watch your portion sizes, too. This an important strategy in keeping track of your nutritional intake and ultimately improving the overall management of weight, metabolic flexibility, and insulin sensitivity.

Here is a list of the best sources of carbs to add to any of the meal plans when you want to carb cycle. I especially recommend starchy vegetables, especially if you are grain-free.

Cooked Starchy Vegetables

Your serving sizes should stay relatively small: ⅓ cup of each, or in the case of sweet potatoes or yams, 1 small piece.

*Beans and lentils
Beets
Carrots
Corn (½ cob)
*Green peas
Parsnips
*Plantain

Pumpkin

*Sweet potato

Winter squash, such as acorn or butternut squash

*Yams

Gluten-Free Grains

Amaranth

Buckwheat

Millet

Oats

Quinoa

*Rice (brown and wild are preferable)

*Sorghum

Teff

*These carbohydrates contain "resistant starches," so called because they resist digestion in the small intestine. When they arrive in the colon, they are fermented by friendly gut bacteria to produce a wide range of benefits: weight loss, blood-sugar and insulin control, reduced appetite, various benefits for digestion. Like fiber, resistant starches act as a prebiotic that feeds the good bacteria in the gut.

Optimization

WEEK 2

Monday

Lunch: Spicy Bison Chili (page 236); green salad with dressing of choice

Dinner: Lamb Shoulder Chops with Olive-Parsley Gremolata (page 232)

Tuesday

Lunch: Beet-Horseradish Deviled Eggs (4 pieces) (page 272), 1 Grain-Free "Golden Milk" Banana Muffin (page 286)

Dinner: Ranch Pork Medallions (page 239), green salad with dressing of choice

Wednesday

Lunch: Egg Roll Bowl (page 284) made with shrimp

Dinner: Chicken Sausage with Sauerkraut and Apple (page 222)

Thursday

Lunch: 4 pieces Beet-Horseradish Deviled Eggs (page 276), 2 spears Prosciutto-Wrapped Asparagus (page 294)

Dinner: Skillet Jambalaya with Cauliflower Rice (page 282)

Friday

Lunch: Cauliflower Gnocchi Caprese (page 277)

Dinner: Spicy Bison Chili (page 236); green salad with dressing of choice

Saturday

Lunch: Brussels Sprout Hash with Bacon and Eggs (page 272)

Dinner: Thai Fish and Vegetable Curry (page 254)

Sunday

Lunch: New-Fashioned Chicken Waldorf Salad (page 264)

Dinner: Spicy Bison Chili (page 236); green salad with dressing of choice

WEEK 3

Monday

Lunch: Shrimp Louie Salad–Stuffed Avocado (page 249), 1 Chocolate Date-"Halvah" Bite (page 289)

Dinner: Lettuce-Wrapped Greek Lamb Meatballs with Tzatziki (page 234)

Tuesday

Lunch: Sesame Zoodles with Vegetables (page 280)

Dinner: Sheet-Pan Roasted Chicken Sausage and Vegetables (page 236)

Wednesday

Lunch: Tuna Puttanesca–Stuffed Tomatoes (page 252), 1 Chocolate Date-"Halvah" Bite (page 289)

Dinner: Flank Steak Teriyaki (page 225), sautéed cauliflower rice, stir-fried broccoli

Thursday

Lunch: Chilled Cucumber-Avocado Soup with Spicy Shrimp (page 248)

Dinner: Sheet-Pan Chicken Fajitas (page 268)

Friday

Lunch: Mini Secret-Ingredient BBQ Meatloaves (page 227), green salad with dressing of choice

Dinner: Fish and Vegetables en Papillote (page 259), 1 Chocolate Date-"Halvah" Bite (page 289)

Saturday

Lunch: Huevos Rancheros Salad (page 271)

Dinner: Crisp Pork Cutlets with Celery-Apple Salad (page 241)

Sunday

Lunch: 1 Pork-Apple Sausage Patty (page 238), 3 scrambled eggs, 1 Glazed Grain-Free Carrot Cake Muffin (page 287)

Dinner: Better-Than-Grandma's Roast Chicken and Vegetables (page 266)

WEEK 4

Monday

Lunch: Asian-inspired chicken salad (using leftover roast chicken)

Dinner: Mussels in Spicy Tomato-Chorizo Broth (page 251)

Tuesday

Lunch: Steak Caesar Salad (page 230), 1 Glazed Grain-Free Carrot Cake Muffin (page 287)

Dinner: Kimchi Shrimp Fried "Rice" (page 247)

Wednesday

Lunch: 1 Pork-Apple Sausage Patty (page 238), 3 eggs scrambled with chopped onion and spinach

Dinner: Cauliflower Gnocchi Caprese (page 277)

Thursday

Lunch: Egg Roll Bowl made with ground turkey (page 284), 1 Glazed Grain-Free Carrot Cake Muffin (page 287)

Dinner: Skirt Steak with Avocado-Horseradish Cream (page 223), sautéed green beans

Friday

Lunch: 1 Pork-Apple Sausage Patty (page 238), 3 eggs scrambled with chopped onion and bell pepper

Dinner: Sheet-Pan Salmon and Broccoli with Lemon-Pepper Butter (page 256)

Saturday

Lunch: New-Fashioned Chicken Waldorf Salad (page 264)

Dinner: Lettuce-Wrapped Greek Lamb Meatballs with Tzatziki (page 234)

Sunday

Lunch: Fennel, Shallot, and Goat Cheese Frittata (page 270); Romesco Dip (page 297) with chopped vegetables

Dinner: Spicy Bison Chili (page 236), green salad with dressing of choice

WEEK 5

Monday

Lunch: 4 pieces "Miso Soup" Deviled Eggs (page 275), 2 spears Prosciutto-Wrapped Asparagus (page 294)

Dinner: Creamy Pesto Chicken-Spinach Casserole (page 250)

Tuesday

Lunch: Spicy Bison Chili (page 236), salad with dressing of choice

Dinner: Sheet-Pan Salmon and Broccoli with Lemon-Pepper Butter (page 256), 1 piece Chocolate-Coconut Freezer Fudge (page 290)

Wednesday

Lunch: Shrimp Louie Salad-Stuffed Avocado (page 249)

Dinner: Flank Steak Teriyaki (page 225), steamed broccoli drizzled with toasted sesame oil

Thursday

Lunch: Creamy Pesto Chicken-Spinach Casserole (page 250)

Dinner: Crisp Pork Cutlets with Celery-Apple Salad (page 241)

Friday

 Lunch: 4 pieces "Miso Soup" Deviled Eggs (page 275), salad with
  dressing of choice

 Dinner: Chipotle-Bacon Scallops (page 258), cauliflower rice, 1 piece
  Chocolate-Coconut Freezer Fudge (page 290)

Saturday

 Lunch: Huevos Rancheros Salad (page 271), 1 Grain-Free "Golden
  Milk" Banana Muffin (page 286)

 Dinner: Thai Fish and Vegetable Curry (page 254)

Sunday

 Lunch: Upgraded Cheeseburgers (page 229), Air Fryer Jicama "Fries"
  with Herbed Mayo (page 295)

 Dinner: Sheet-Pan Roasted Chicken Sausage and Vegetables
  (page 263), 1 piece Chocolate-Coconut Freezer Fudge (page 290)

Modification

WEEK 6

Monday

 Lunch: Dairy-Free Spaghetti Squash "Alfredo" (page 278) topped
  with 4 ounces protein of choice

 Dinner: Vietnamese Caramel Pork (page 240)

Tuesday

 Lunch: Sesame Zoodles with Vegetables (page 280)

 Dinner: Mussels in Spicy Tomato-Chorizo Broth (page 251),
  1 Chocolate Date-"Halvah" Bite (page 289)

Wednesday

 Lunch: Tuna Puttanesca–Stuffed Tomatoes (page 252), 1 Glazed
  Grain-Free Carrot Cake Muffin (page 287)

 Dinner: Lettuce-Wrapped Greek Lamb Meatballs with Tzatziki
  (page 234)

Thursday

 Lunch: Brussels Sprout Hash with Bacon and Eggs (page 272)

 Dinner: Cauliflower Gnocchi Caprese (page 277)

Friday

> Lunch: Beet-Horseradish Deviled Eggs (page 276), green salad with dressing of choice; 1 Glazed Grain-Free Carrot Cake Muffin (page 287)
>
> Dinner: Better-Than-Grandma's Roast Chicken and Vegetables (page 266)

Saturday

> Lunch: Asian-inspired chicken salad (using leftover roast chicken; see Got Leftovers?, p. 267)
>
> Dinner: Salmon Cakes (page 253), green salad with dressing of choice

Sunday

> Lunch: Fennel, Shallot, and Goat Cheese Frittata (page 270), 1 Chocolate Date-"Halvah" Bite (page 289)
>
> Dinner: Chicken Sausage with Sauerkraut and Apple (page 222)

Chapter 14

. . . .

The IF:45 Recipes

Just because you are following a nutrition program does not mean that you have to give up the pleasures of enjoying delicious food! My IF:45 plan recipes are carefully designed to give you the right macros to have during your feeding window, but they are also full of flavor and satisfying. They're easy to prepare and make wonderful leftovers, too. Each recipe has a macronutrient count so you know exactly how many grams of protein, carbohydrates, and fat you're eating.

BEEF RECIPES

Skirt Steak with Avocado-Horseradish Cream

Skirt steak is a very ropy and tender cut. It cooks quickly, so it's great for busy weeknights. If it's cooked more than medium-rare it gets really tough, so it's not the cut for you if you prefer medium or beyond. But the avocado-horseradish cream would go well on other cuts, so use it on your fave.

PREP: 15 minutes
COOK: 15 minutes
SERVES: 4

Steak:

  1½ *pounds skirt steak*
  Fine sea salt and freshly ground black pepper
  2 *tablespoons avocado oil*

Cream:

  1 *ripe avocado*
  1 *tablespoon prepared horseradish*
  1 *tablespoon extra-virgin olive oil*
  2 *teaspoons lemon juice*
  ½ *teaspoon garlic powder*
  ½ *teaspoon coconut aminos*
  Fine sea salt and freshly ground black pepper

1. Make the steak: If steak is in one long piece, cut it into two or three pieces so it fits in the pan. Place a large cast-iron or heavy-bottomed skillet over high heat until hot. Pat the steak dry very thoroughly; season with salt and pepper. Swirl the avocado oil in the skillet and add the steak. Cook for 3 to 4 minutes, until just seared and browned on the bottom. Flip and sear on the other side, 2 to 4 minutes longer (an instant read thermometer stuck into the thickest part should read 130°F). Transfer to a cutting board; cover to keep warm, and let rest for 10 minutes.

2. While the steak is resting, make the cream: Pit and peel the avocado and place in the bowl of a food processor. Add the horseradish, olive oil, lemon juice, garlic powder, and coconut aminos. Process until smooth. Taste and season with salt and pepper. (This should yield about ⅔ cup.)

3. Slice the steak against the grain and serve with 1 to 2 tablespoons avocado cream.

PER SERVING: 541 calories, 35g protein, 29g fat, 4g carbohydrates, 3g fiber

NOTE:
....

You may need to cook the steak in batches. Add more oil to the skillet between batches if needed. Cover the cooked steak to keep it warm while you cook the rest and slice it all before serving.

If you have leftover avocado cream, cover and refrigerate it. It's delicious alongside any protein, or use it as a dip for cut-up vegetables.

How to Use Avocado Oil

I love to cook with avocado oil. Like its source, the luscious avocado, avocado oil is a heart-healthy monounsaturated fat rich in vitamins A, B₁, B₂, D and E—all great for things like your cells, waistline, skin, and even hair. This oil is also a powerful antioxidant that fights disease-causing free radicals.

Besides its health benefits, avocado oil tastes delicious—light, fresh, and perfect for most foods. It can be easily swapped with olive oil, coconut oil, or sesame oil with tasty results.

Avocado oil has the highest smoke point of cooking oils, from 470°F to 500°F, making it by far the safest oil for high-heat cooking. This is important because some oils, when cooked at a high heat, can burn, break down on a chemical level, and become toxic. You don't have to worry about this with avocado oil.

This amazing oil is versatile, too. You can use it in your salad dressings or homemade mayonnaise, drizzle it over hummus, swirl it in soups, sauté veggies, or use it as part of a marinade.

Flank Steak Teriyaki

Teriyaki sauce is one of those things we usually just automatically buy ready-made, but once you've made your own, you won't go back. It's so easy, and the result is so much better. Make some extra and drizzle it on any protein or vegetables you like.

PREP: 15 minutes
MARINATE: 4 to 8 hours
COOK: 20 minutes
SERVES: 4

> 1 teaspoon arrowroot
> 2 tablespoons avocado oil
> 4 garlic cloves, minced (1 tablespoon plus 1 teaspoon)
> 2 tablespoons minced fresh ginger
> ⅔ cup coconut aminos
> 2 tablespoons mirin
> 1½ teaspoons raw honey
> 1 teaspoon orange zest
> Freshly ground black pepper
> 1½ pounds flank steak, patted dry
> Fine sea salt

1. Mix the arrowroot with 1 tablespoon water in a small bowl until dissolved. Warm 1 tablespoon of the avocado oil in a small saucepan over medium-low heat. Add the garlic and ginger; sauté until fragrant, about 1 minute. Whisk in the coconut aminos, mirin, honey, and orange zest. Whisk the arrowroot mixture into the sauce. Bring the sauce to a boil, then reduce the heat to low and cook, whisking, until the sauce has thickened, about 1 minute. Transfer to a small bowl; taste and season with pepper. Let cool. (This should yield 1 cup.) Pour half of the sauce into a cup, cover, and refrigerate. When you serve the steak with the sauce, you can drizzle on at least 1 and often 2 tablespoons, which should use up most if not all the sauce.
2. Place the other half of the sauce into a large resealable bag. Add the steak (cut it into 2 pieces if it's very long). Seal the bag and turn it over a few times to coat the steak with the sauce. Refrigerate for at least 4 and up to 8 hours.
3. Allow the steak to stand at room temperature for 20 minutes. Heat a large cast-iron or heavy-bottomed skillet over high heat until very

hot. Swirl the remaining 1 tablespoon oil in the pan. Season the steak lightly with salt and sear on one side for 3 to 4 minutes. Using tongs, carefully turn the steak and cook until seared on the other side and an instant-read thermometer stuck into the thickest part reads 130°F for medium-rare, 3 to 4 minutes longer. Transfer the steak to a cutting board, tent with foil, and let rest for 5 to 10 minutes. Gently rewarm the reserved sauce in a small saucepan over low heat, stirring.

4. Slice the steak thinly against the grain. Divide among 4 plates and serve, passing the reserved sauce on the side.

PER SERVING: 438 calories, 36g protein, 19g fat, 18g carbohydrates, 0g fiber

Make it plant-based
Use the sauce on a plant-based protein.

Mini Secret-Ingredient BBQ Meatloaves

Just saying the word "liver" makes some people scrunch up their faces, but the thing is, your grandma was right: It's one of the most nutrient-dense foods you can eat. If you or someone in your family is dead-set against eating it, these little meatloaf muffins are for you. Liver is minced, along with bacon, and essentially hidden within lots of ground beef, spices, and barbecue sauce. You don't taste liver—just rich, satisfying meatloaf. And since the liver is so healthy, a little goes a long way.

PREP: 20 minutes
COOK: 25 minutes
YIELD: 12 mini meatloaves

> *Olive or avocado oil, for greasing the pan*
> *1¼ pounds ground beef (preferably 100% grass-fed)*
> *2 ounces uncured bacon, minced*
> *2 ounces beef liver, minced*

1 large egg, beaten

¾ cup pork panko (such as Bacon's Heir)

2 teaspoons garlic powder

2 teaspoons dried oregano

1 teaspoon onion powder

½ teaspoon fine sea salt

¼ teaspoon freshly ground black pepper

¼ cup no-sugar-added barbecue sauce (such as True Made Foods)

1. Preheat the oven to 350°F. Lightly brush the wells of a 12-cup nonstick muffin tin with oil.
2. In a large bowl, combine the beef, bacon, liver, egg, panko, garlic powder, oregano, onion powder, salt, and pepper. Use your hands to gently but thoroughly mix until all the ingredients are well combined.
3. Divide the mixture among the muffin cups (an ice cream scoop is useful here). Use your fingers to lightly press the mixture in so it's level. Place 1 teaspoon of barbecue sauce on each meatloaf, spreading to cover the top.
4. Bake for 20 to 25 minutes, until the meatloaves are cooked through (an instant read thermometer stuck into the center of a meatloaf should read 160°F). Let cool for 5 minutes in the pan before removing. Serve hot, or let cool, cover, and refrigerate to serve later (meatloaves will keep in the refrigerator for up to 4 days).

NOTE:

Ask your butcher if they'll make you a custom grind, with 80% beef, 10% bacon, and 10% liver. You might have to order a minimum (my butcher requires 3 pounds); just double the meatloaf recipe or freeze some for later. The mix makes delicious burgers, too.

PER SERVING (2 MEATLOAVES): 313 calories, 30g protein, 20g fat, 3g carbohydrates, 1g fiber

Upgraded Cheeseburgers

If you thought nothing could make a good old-fashioned cheeseburger
any better, get ready: With grass-fed beef, a quick tangy sauce, a good-
quality cheese, and caramelized onion, all on top of a toasted grain-free
cauliflower round, these burgers not only taste amazing, they'll leave you
feeling great afterward, too.

PREP: 15 minutes
COOK: 30 minutes
SERVES: 4

Sauce:

¼ cup mayonnaise

2 tablespoons no-sugar-added ketchup

2 tablespoons minced half-sour pickle

½ teaspoon coconut aminos

¼ teaspoon hot sauce

¼ teaspoon smoked paprika

Fine sea salt and freshly ground black pepper

Burgers:

1 tablespoon ghee

1 yellow onion, halved, thinly sliced

Fine sea salt and freshly ground black pepper

1½ pounds ground beef

4 slices cheddar cheese (preferably sheep's milk)

4 cauliflower rounds, such as Outer Aisle, toasted

1. Make the sauce: In a small bowl, whisk together the mayonnaise,
   ketchup, pickle, coconut aminos, hot sauce, and paprika. Taste and
   season with salt and pepper. (This will yield about ½ cup.)
2. Melt the ghee in a large skillet over medium heat. Add the onion and
   season with salt. Cook for 15 to 18 minutes, stirring occasionally,
   until the onion is golden brown, watching carefully and stirring

more often toward the end of the cooking time to prevent burning. Transfer to a bowl; cover to keep warm.

3. Divide the ground beef into 4 portions; shape into 4-inch-wide patties. Warm the same skillet over high heat until hot. Season the patties generously with salt and pepper and place in the skillet. Cook for about 3 minutes, until seared on the bottom. Flip and cook on the other side for 3 to 5 minutes longer, until seared and an instant-read thermometer inserted into the center reads 145°F for medium-rare. Add a slice of cheese on top for the last minute to melt it.

4. Place a cauliflower round on each of 4 plates. Top each with 1 tablespoon sauce and one-fourth of onions and serve. (Pass the remaining sauce on the side, if desired.)

PER SERVING: 595 calories, 45g protein, 44g fat, 6g carbohydrates, 1g fiber

Steak Caesar Salad

You don't need cheese or croutons to make a savory, delicious Caesar salad. Hemp hearts, a complete protein, give the dressing body, and the texture of Parmesan and roasted sunflower seeds sprinkled on top bring the saltiness and crunch. New York strip steak on top makes it a complete meal, but grilled chicken, shrimp, or any other protein you have on hand can fill in.

PREP: 20 minutes
COOK: 15 minutes
SERVES: 4

Dressing:

4 tablespoons extra-virgin olive oil
3 jarred or tinned anchovy filets
2 garlic cloves, minced
½ teaspoon lemon zest
2 tablespoons lemon juice

2 tablespoons hemp hearts

1 large egg yolk

Fine sea salt and freshly ground black pepper

Salad:

1½ pounds New York strip steak (1½ inches thick), patted dry

Fine sea salt and freshly ground black pepper

1 tablespoon avocado oil

2 tablespoons unsalted butter

3 garlic cloves, smashed

1 large or 2 medium heads romaine (about 14 ounces), chopped (about 8 cups)

4 teaspoons roasted, salted sunflower seeds

1. Make the dressing: In a small, unheated skillet, combine 1 tablespoon olive oil, the anchovies, and garlic. Place over low heat and cook undisturbed until the mixture begins to sizzle. Allow it to sizzle for 30 seconds, then transfer to the bowl of a small food processor. Add the lemon zest and juice, hemp hearts, and egg yolk; process until smooth. Add the remaining 3 tablespoons oil. Blend until well combined, thickened, and emulsified. Taste and season with salt and pepper. (You can make the dressing 1 day ahead; keep covered and refrigerated. Whisk before using.)

2. Let the steak stand at room temperature for 30 minutes. Heat a large cast-iron or other heavy-bottomed skillet over medium-high heat until very hot. Season the steak all over generously with salt and pepper. Swirl the avocado oil in the skillet and add the steak. Cook for 3 to 4 minutes, until seared on one side. Flip the steak and cook for 3 to 4 minutes longer, until seared on the other side. Reduce the heat to medium and add the butter and garlic (the butter will melt quickly). Baste the steak with the garlic butter by spooning it over the steak several times. Continue to cook for 4 to 7 minutes, turning the steak a couple of times and basting, until a meat thermometer stuck into the thickest part reads 135°F for medium-rare. Transfer the steak to a cutting board; cover, and let rest for at least 5 minutes.

3. Place the lettuce in a large bowl. Add half of the dressing (about
   ⅓ cup) and toss. Toss in more dressing, if desired. Divide among
   4 shallow bowls; sprinkle each with 1 teaspoon sunflower seeds.
   Slice the steak against the grain. Top each salad with one-fourth of
   the steak and serve.

PER SERVING: 351 calories, 17g protein, 27g fat, 7g carbohydrates,
2g fiber

NOTE:
If using raw egg yolk is a concern, use pasteurized eggs.

Make it plant-based:
Replace the steak with drained canned beans or lentils and drizzle on a
bottled vegan Caesar dressing.

LAMB RECIPES

Lamb Shoulder Chops with Olive-Parsley Gremolata

Lamb shoulder blade chops are a fantastic way to enjoy lamb. This cut is far
less expensive than delicate lamb rib chops, but they're loaded with flavor,
and though they're often braised, they actually work beautifully seared in a
skillet, as we do here. The simple marinade gives them extra depth. Make
the gremolata in advance, if you like, so dinner is on the table fast.

PREP: 20 minutes (plus up to 8 hours marinating time)
COOK: 20 minutes
SERVES: 4

Chops:
   2 tablespoons avocado oil
   3 garlic cloves, minced (1 tablespoon)
   1 teaspoon dried oregano
   ½ teaspoon fine sea salt

¼ teaspoon freshly ground black pepper

4 lamb shoulder blade chops (8 to 10 ounces each), pat dry

Gremolata:

1½ tablespoons extra-virgin olive oil

1 garlic clove, minced (1 teaspoon)

½ cup mixed green and black olives, pitted and chopped

2 tablespoons chopped fresh flat-leaf parsley

½ teaspoon lemon zest

1 teaspoons lemon juice

Pinch crushed red pepper flakes

Fine sea salt and freshly grated black pepper

1. Make the chops: In a bowl, combine the avocado oil, garlic, oregano, salt, and pepper. Place the chops in a large resealable bag. Add the oil mixture, seal the bag, and turn over a few times to coat the chops with the marinade. Allow the chops to marinate at room temperature for 30 minutes, or refrigerate in the marinade for up to 8 hours. (If the chops are refrigerated, let them stand at room temperature for 30 minutes before cooking.)

2. Make the gremolata: Combine the olive oil and garlic in a small unheated skillet. Place over medium-low heat; cook until the mixture begins to sizzle. Allow it to sizzle for 30 seconds, then transfer to a medium bowl to cool. When it has cooled, add the olives, parsley, lemon zest and juice, and red pepper flakes; stir to combine. Taste and season with pepper. (You can make the gremolata up to 1 day ahead; cover and refrigerate.)

3. Preheat a large cast-iron skillet over medium-high heat until very hot. Remove the chops from the marinade and season with salt and pepper to taste. Place the chops in the skillet and cook for 3 to 5 minutes per side (depending on the thickness), until well seared on both sides and a meat thermometer stuck into the thickest part away from the bone reads 130°F. Transfer to a cutting board, cover loosely with foil, and let rest for 5 minutes before serving with gremolata.

PER SERVING: 579 calories, 29g protein, 50g fat, 3g carbohydrates, 0g fiber

NOTE:

If you have two skillets, you can cook all the chops at once. If not, cook them two at a time and keep the first ones warm while you cook the second batch.

Lettuce-Wrapped Greek Lamb Meatballs with Tzatziki

Zaatar gives these lamb meatballs that something extra. This Middle Eastern spice blend—usually made with dried thyme, oregano, sumac, and toasted sesame seeds—is worth keeping in the pantry, as it enlivens meat, fish, chicken, and vegetables beautifully. Meatballs are a great place to start if you're less familiar cooking with lamb; they're easy and a crowd pleaser. The tzatziki is a must to bring the dish together.

PREP: 30 minutes
COOK: 20 minutes
SERVES: 4

Tzatziki:

    ½ English cucumber
    Fine sea salt
    1 tablespoon extra-virgin olive oil
    2 garlic cloves, minced (2 teaspoons)
    ¾ cup full-fat Greek yogurt
    1½ tablespoons lemon juice
    2 teaspoons minced fresh mint
    Freshly ground black pepper

Meatballs:

    1 pound ground lamb
    3 tablespoons cassava flour
    2 tablespoons extra-virgin olive oil
    2 teaspoons garlic powder

2 teaspoons dried oregano
2 teaspoons zaatar
1 tablespoon minced fresh mint
½ teaspoon fine sea salt
¼ teaspoon freshly ground black pepper
Olive oil cooking spray
1 cup halved cherry or grape tomatoes, for serving
¼ cup chopped pitted kalamata or oil-cured olives, for serving
Bibb lettuce leaves, for serving

1. Make the tzatziki: Grate the cucumber on the large holes of a box grater. Place in a fine-mesh sieve. Sprinkle with ¼ teaspoon salt; toss. Let stand for 10 minutes. In a small, unheated skillet, combine the olive oil and garlic. Place over low heat and cook until the mixture sizzles. Allow it to sizzle for 30 seconds, then transfer to a medium bowl.

2. Press the cucumber to remove some of the water, then roll it up in a clean kitchen towel and wring out as much water as possible. Transfer to the bowl with the garlic mixture. Add the yogurt, lemon juice, and mint; fold together until well incorporated. Taste and season with salt and pepper. (This will yield about 1 cup. You can make the tzatziki up to 1 day ahead; keep covered in the fridge. Stir before using.)

3. Make the meatballs: Preheat the oven to 350°F; line a baking sheet with parchment paper.

4. In a large bowl, combine the lamb, cassava, olive oil, garlic powder, oregano, zaatar, mint, salt, and pepper. Using your hands, gently but thoroughly mix until all the ingredients are well combined. Divide into 12 portions (a small ice cream scoop is useful here); roll into balls and place on the baking sheet. Mist the meatballs with cooking spray. Bake for 15 to 18 minutes, until cooked through.

5. Place the tomatoes and olives in separate bowls; place the lettuce on a plate. Serve the meatballs and tzatziki and let everyone make their own lettuce wraps.

PER SERVING: 508 calories, 30g protein, 35g fat, 20g carbohydrates, 3g fiber

PORK RECIPES

Spicy Bison Chili

Chili is better if it's had time for the flavor to develop. So if possible, make this the day before you're going to serve it and refrigerate it overnight, then rewarm it the next day. If it needs something after you've added the lime juice and seasoned with salt and pepper, try stirring in some honey—sometimes a small hit of sweetness is just the thing to brighten the flavor.

PREP: 30 minutes
COOK: 1 hour
YIELD: About 9 cups

    1 tablespoon bacon fat or avocado oil
    8 ounces spicy pork sausage, casings removed
    1 large onion, chopped (about 2½ cups)
    1 large jalapeño, seeds removed, minced (about ⅓ cup)
    2 large ribs celery, diced (about ¾ cup)
    1 medium red bell pepper, seeded and diced (about 1 cup)
    Fine sea salt and freshly ground black pepper
    3 garlic cloves, minced (1 tablespoon)
    1½ pounds ground bison
    1 tablespoon chili powder
    1 tablespoon dried oregano
    1½ teaspoons ground cumin
    ½ teaspoon smoked paprika
    ¼ teaspoon ground cinnamon
    1 15-ounce can fire-roasted diced tomatoes
    2 tablespoons tomato paste

1 tablespoon coconut aminos

1 cup beef or chicken bone broth

1 tablespoon lime juice or cider vinegar

¼ teaspoon honey (optional)

Toppings: Diced avocado, shredded cheddar, sour cream, diced radishes,
    cilantro, or other toppings (optional)

1. Melt the bacon fat in a large Dutch oven over medium heat. Add the
   sausage and cook for 5 to 7 minutes, breaking it up with a wooden
   spoon and stirring, until the sausage is cooked through and golden
   in spots and the fat has rendered. Add the onion, jalapeño, celery,
   and bell pepper. Sprinkle with salt and pepper and cook for 6 to
   8 minutes, stirring, until tender. Add the garlic; sauté for about
   1 minute, until fragrant.

2. Add the bison. Season generously with salt and pepper and cook for
   6 to 8 minutes, breaking up the meat and stirring with a wooden
   spoon, until cooked through. Add the chili powder, oregano, cumin,
   paprika, and cinnamon; cook for 1 to 2 minutes, stirring, until the
   spices are well incorporated and fragrant.

3. Add the tomatoes, tomato paste, coconut aminos, and broth; cook,
   stirring and pulling up browned bits off the bottom of the pot. Bring
   just to a light boil, then reduce the heat to low and bring to a
   simmer. Cover and simmer for 30 minutes.

4. Stir the lime juice and optional honey into the chili. Taste and season
   with salt and pepper. Serve with the toppings, if desired, or let cool,
   cover, and refrigerate to serve later. Rewarm on the stove over
   medium-low heat.

PER SERVING (1 CUP): 378 calories, 59g protein, 12g fat,
9g carbohydrates, 2g fiber

Make it plant-based:
Use plant-based sausage and replace the ground bison with drained
canned beans and/or lentils.

Pork-Apple Sausage Patties

Serving sausage you made from scratch gives you instant credibility as a cook; no need to tell anyone how easy it is. You can make the patties up to a day in advance and keep them covered and refrigerated, if you like. Or cook them, let cool, cover, and refrigerate to serve later. Rewarm them gently in a skillet or covered on a tray in your toaster oven.

PREP: 10 minutes
COOK: 8 minutes per batch
YIELD: 8 patties

> 1 pound ground pork
> 1 small tart apple (such as Granny Smith), peeled, cored, and shredded on a
>   box grater (about ½ cup)
> 2 teaspoons minced fresh sage
> ½ teaspoon garlic powder
> ¾ teaspoon fine sea salt
> ¼ teaspoon freshly ground black pepper

1. In a large bowl, combine the pork, apple, sage, garlic powder, salt, and pepper. Use your fingers to gently but thoroughly mix well. Divide into 8 portions; form into ¼-inch-thick patties (they'll be about 2½ inches in diameter).
2. Warm a large nonstick skillet over medium heat. Add the patties and cook for 5 to 8 minutes total, flipping halfway through, until cooked through and lightly browned (don't overcrowd the pan; work in batches if needed). Serve hot.

PER SERVING (1 PATTY): 155 calories, 10g protein, 11g fat, 4g carbohydrates, 1g fiber

Ranch Pork Medallions

Brining the pork tenderloin in buttermilk spiked with spices gives these medallions that tangy, creamy ranch flavor. If the weather permits, you can grill the medallions instead of pan-frying. A drizzle of Buffalo wing sauce, such as Frank's RedHot, is delicious on these if you like some heat.

PREP: 15 minutes
COOK: 10 minutes
SERVES: 4

> 1 tablespoon dried parsley
> 1 tablespoon garlic powder
> 2 teaspoons dried chives
> 2 teaspoons onion powder
> 1½ teaspoons dried dill
> ¼ teaspoon sweet paprika
> 2 cups low-fat buttermilk
> 2 teaspoons honey
> 1 tablespoon fine sea salt
> ½ teaspoon freshly ground black pepper
> 1 1½-pound pork tenderloin
> 2 tablespoons ghee or avocado oil

1. In a large bowl, combine the parsley, garlic powder, chives, onion powder, dill, and paprika; stir with a fork to mix well. This should yield about 5 tablespoons. Remove half and reserve the remaining 2½ tablespoons (cover and refrigerate). Whisk the buttermilk, honey, salt, and pepper into the large bowl with the remaining spice mixture.

2. Trim any excess fat off the pork. If there's a thin, silvery membrane on it, remove it by slicing it with a paring knife and pulling it off with your fingers (use the knife to slice off the ends of the membrane, if needed). Cut the pork crosswise into ½-inch-thick

pieces. Pat them dry and add them to the bowl with the buttermilk mixture. Cover and refrigerate for at least 4 hours or up to overnight.

3. When you're ready to cook the meat, remove the pork pieces from the brine and wipe any excess brine from the pork. Discard the brine. Cut the pork into ½-inch-thick slices. Use the side of your chef's knife to press down on the slices to flatten them to ¼-inch thickness. Season with salt and sprinkle with the reserved spice mixture, pressing to adhere.

4. Melt the ghee in a large skillet over medium-high heat. Place the medallions in the hot skillet and cook for 1 to 3 minutes per side, until seared and no longer pink inside. (Do not overcrowd the pan; work in batches if needed, adding more ghee between batches.) Cover to keep warm; let rest for 5 minutes. Serve.

NOTE:

If you have leftover buttermilk and no immediate use for it, you can freeze it. If you plan to use it all at once, freeze it in its container. If you'll use smaller amounts, freeze it in an ice cube tray or silicone muffin molds, then pop out and place in a freezer bag.

PER SERVING: 271 calories, 36g protein, 11g fat, 8g carbohydrates, 1g fiber

Vietnamese Caramel Pork

"Caramel" may sound like a strange thing to have with pork, but once you've tasted this, you'll get why that's the perfect name for it. The coconut sugar caramelizes beautifully, elevating the garlic, ginger, and pork flavors. Mint and basil add brightness to the finished dish. My favorite way to eat this is wrapped up in lettuce leaves (or straight out of the skillet; don't tell anyone).

PREP: 15 minutes
COOK: 20 minutes
SERVES: 4 (can be doubled)

2 tablespoons avocado oil

6 scallions, white and light green parts sliced on a diagonal (¾ cup)

1 tablespoon minced fresh ginger

2 garlic cloves, minced (2 teaspoons)

2 teaspoons drained jarred lemongrass, minced (optional)

1 small red or green chili pepper (such as a Thai or Fresno chili), seeded and thinly sliced

Fine sea salt

1 pound ground pork

5 tablespoons coconut sugar

2½ tablespoons fish sauce

Bibb lettuce leaves, cooked rice, or cauliflower rice, for serving

Chopped fresh mint and Thai basil, for serving (optional)

1. Warm the avocado oil in a large skillet over medium-high heat. Add the scallions, ginger, garlic, lemongrass (if using), and red chili; season with a pinch of salt. Cook for 1 to 2 minutes, stirring, until fragrant. Add the pork; cook for 2 to 3 minutes, stirring with a wooden spoon, until cooked partway and broken up.
2. Stir in the coconut sugar and fish sauce until well combined. Spread the mixture in the skillet and let it cook undisturbed for 2 minutes. Stir, spread it out again, and let it cook undisturbed for 30 seconds to 1 minute to allow the mixture to caramelize. Repeat for 5 to 7 minutes longer, until the meat is deep golden, fragrant, and well caramelized.
3. Serve hot with lettuce, rice, or cauliflower rice. Add mint and/or Thai basil, if desired.

PER SERVING: 438 calories, 21g protein, 29g fat, 26g carbohydrates, 1g fiber

Crisp Pork Cutlets with Celery-Apple Salad

Pork tenderloin dredged in pork panko and pan-fried—now that's indulgent, in the best way. A light salad with endive, celery, apple, fresh parsley, and a little bit of dried dates is a perfect foil to the rich meat. You could make this dish with thin chicken cutlets instead of pork, if you prefer.

PREP: 30 minutes
COOK: 6 minutes per batch
SERVES: 4

Salad:

2 heads endive, halved lengthwise, thinly sliced (about 3 cups)
4 ribs celery, thinly sliced on a diagonal (about 1¾ cups)
1 medium apple, cored and chopped (about 1½ cups)
⅓ cup fresh flat-leaf parsley leaves
¼ cup pitted dried dates, finely chopped
1 tablespoon extra-virgin olive oil
1 tablespoon lemon juice
Fine sea salt and freshly ground black pepper

Pork:

1 1¼- to 1½-pound pork tenderloin, trimmed
Fine sea salt and freshly ground black pepper
1 large egg
¾ cup pork panko
2 tablespoons arrowroot
½ teaspoon garlic powder
¼ teaspoon onion powder
¼ teaspoon smoked paprika
Avocado oil, for frying
Lemon wedges, for serving (optional)

1. Preheat the oven to 200°F; line a rimmed baking sheet with a cooling rack and place in the oven.
2. Make the salad: In a medium bowl, combine the endive, celery, apple, parsley, and dates. Drizzle with the olive oil and lemon juice; gently toss. Season with salt and pepper; toss again.

3. Make the pork cutlets: Cut the pork into ½-inch-thick slices. Using the side of a chef's knife, press down to flatten the pork into ¼-inch-thick slices. Pat dry and season with salt and pepper.

4. In a shallow bowl, beat the egg. In a separate shallow bowl, whisk together the panko, arrowroot, garlic powder, onion powder, and paprika. Warm a ¼-inch layer of avocado oil in a large skillet over medium-high heat.

5. Dip the pork pieces in the egg, shake off the excess, then dredge in panko mixture, pressing to adhere. Repeat with the remaining pork. Add a few pieces of breaded pork to the skillet (do not overcrowd the skillet) and cook for 2 to 3 minutes, until golden on one side. Carefully flip and cook for 2 to 3 minutes longer, until golden on both sides and cooked through. Transfer the cooked cutlets to the oven to keep warm and repeat with the remaining cutlets, adding more oil between batches.

6. Divide the salad among 4 plates. Divide the pork among the plates. Serve with lemon wedges on the side.

PER SERVING: 541 calories, 55g protein, 23g fat, 26g carbohydrates, 4g fiber

NOTE:
....
This salad would go nicely with chicken or fish, too. If the entrée isn't crunchy like these pork chops, add a crunchy element to the salad, like dry roasted, salted pistachios.

Baby Kale and Sausage Spaghetti Squash Bake

If you're in the mood for lasagna but not all the carbs and loads of cheese, this dish is for you. Layers of spaghetti squash stand in for noodles, and a bit of goat cheese is all you need for creaminess. With plenty of vegetables and savory sausage, this is a satisfying one-dish meal the whole family will love.

PREP: 20 minutes
COOK: 1 hour 15 minutes
SERVES: 4

> 1 medium spaghetti squash (about 2½ pounds)
> 2 tablespoons extra-virgin olive oil
> Fine sea salt and freshly ground black pepper
> 1 pound sweet or hot Italian sausage, casings removed
> 1 medium yellow onion, chopped (about 1½ cups)
> 3 garlic cloves, minced (1 tablespoon)
> 5 ounces baby kale, chopped
> 1½ cups jarred marinara sauce
> 4 ounces soft goat cheese, crumbled

1. Preheat the oven to 400°F; line a large baking sheet with parchment paper. Grease an 8-inch square baking dish.
2. Place the squash on a sturdy cutting board. Using a sharp chef's knife, slice off the rounded bottom part and stem end of the squash. Turn the squash so that it sits flat on the sliced-off bottom. Cut through the middle of the squash to halve it lengthwise. Using a tablespoon, scrape out the seeds.
3. Brush the inside of the squash with 1 tablespoon of the olive oil; season with salt and pepper. Place the squash cut-side down on the baking sheet. Roast for 45 to 50 minutes, until the squash is tender and easily pierced with a knife. Carefully turn over and let cool slightly.
4. Warm the remaining 1 tablespoon oil in a large skillet over medium heat. Add the sausage and cook for 7 to 9 minutes, stirring and breaking up the meat with a wooden spoon, until the meat is cooked through and browned in spots. Using a slotted spoon, transfer to a large bowl. Add the onion to the skillet, season with salt and pepper, and cook for 6 to 8 minutes, stirring, until tender. Add the garlic; sauté for 1 minute, until fragrant. Add the kale a handful at a time, seasoning with salt, and cook for 3 to 4 minutes, stirring, until the kale is wilted. Add the mixture to the bowl with the sausage.

5. Using a fork, scrape the strands of spaghetti squash out of each half. (This will yield about 3½ cups.) Spread half of the squash in the baking dish. Top with half of the sausage mixture. Spread half of the sauce over; sprinkle with half of the goat cheese. Repeat the layers, ending with the goat cheese. Bake for 20 to 25 minutes, until warmed through and bubbling. Serve hot.

PER SERVING: 468 calories, 26g protein, 26g fat, 34g carbohydrates, 7g fiber

NOTE:
You can make elements of this dish in advance, so all you have to do at dinnertime is assemble and bake. Cook the squash in advance, scrape out the strands, cover, and refrigerate. Cook the sausage-onion-kale mixture; store in a separate covered bowl in the fridge. Give it a few extra minutes in the oven to warm through.

Make it plant-based:
You can leave out the sausage; add chopped sautéed mushrooms instead to bulk up the dish.

Classic Pulled Pork

Making pulled pork in a slow cooker has become a default, but I advocate for the Dutch oven. Yes, it's a little bit more hands-on—but really, just a bit, and the results are so much better. The meat shreds beautifully, it's tender without being soggy, and it has so much flavor. It's a guaranteed crowd favorite, whether you pile it on a salad, have it on a low-carb bun, or top it with a runny fried egg.

PREP: 20 minutes
COOK: 3 hours 15 minutes
YIELD: About 8 cups

> 3 tablespoons coconut sugar
> 2 teaspoons garlic powder

2 teaspoons dried oregano

1 teaspoon fine sea salt

1 teaspoon smoked paprika

1 teaspoon sweet paprika

½ teaspoon freshly ground black pepper

½ teaspoon chili powder

4 pounds boneless pork shoulder, excess fat trimmed, cut into 2-inch pieces, patted dry

2 tablespoons avocado oil

½ cup chicken bone broth

No-sugar barbecue sauce, for serving (optional)

1. Preheat the oven to 300°F.
2. In a large bowl, whisk together the coconut sugar, garlic powder, oregano, salt, both paprikas, pepper, and chili powder. Add the pork and toss until the meat is coated with the spices.
3. Warm the avocado oil in a Dutch oven over medium-high heat. Add the pork and cook for 3 to 5 minutes, until seared on all sides, turning a few times with tongs. (Do not crowd the pan; if all the pieces don't fit in a single layer, work in batches, adding more oil between batches.)
4. Once the pork pieces are seared, add any reserved pieces back (pour in any juices that have collected as well). Pour in the broth, cover, and transfer to the oven. Bake for 2½ to 3 hours, until the meat is cooked through and shreds easily, the liquid has evaporated, and the fat has rendered. (If there's still too much liquid left after 3 hours, uncover and cook for 15 to 20 minutes longer.) Shred the meat and stir. Taste and season with additional salt and pepper, if needed. Eat right away, or let cool, cover, and refrigerate to use later. Serve with barbecue sauce, if desired.

PER SERVING (1 CUP): 375 calories, 55g protein, 12g fat, 7g carbohydrates, 1g fiber

FISH/SHELLFISH RECIPES

Kimchi Shrimp Fried "Rice"

A takeout favorite is transformed into a vegetable-rich, gut-health-supportive nutrition powerhouse. Cauliflower rice stands in for the starchier kind, fresh garlic and ginger add a ton of flavor and anti-inflammatory benefits, shrimp lends protein. Kimchi, a Korean spicy dish made with fermented cabbage and lots of chilies, adds heat. And it all comes together as quickly as ordering in.

PREP: 15 minutes
COOK: 15 minutes
SERVES: 4

1 tablespoon unsalted butter
1¼ pounds medium or large shrimp, peeled and deveined
Fine sea salt and freshly ground black pepper
1 tablespoon avocado oil
6 scallions, trimmed, white and light green parts sliced on a diagonal (about
     ¾ cup; reserve dark green parts for garnish)
1½ tablespoons minced fresh ginger
1 12-ounce package frozen cauliflower rice
2 tablespoons coconut aminos
2 cups chopped drained kimchi
2 tablespoons toasted sesame oil

1. Melt the butter in a large skillet over medium heat. Add the shrimp, season with salt and pepper, and cook for 3 to 4 minutes, until opaque. Transfer to a bowl; cover to keep warm.
2. Warm the avocado oil in the same skillet. Add the scallions and ginger; season with a pinch of salt. Cook for about 1 minute, stirring, until fragrant and tender. Add the cauliflower rice, season with salt and pepper, raise the heat to medium-high, and cook for 4 to

6 minutes, stirring, until warmed through and tender. Stir in the coconut aminos; sauté for about 1 minute, until liquid cooks off.

3. Add the shrimp back to the skillet; toss for 1 minute. Add the kimchi; toss for a few seconds just to take the chill off the kimchi, then remove from the heat. Drizzle with the sesame oil, sprinkle with dark scallion greens, and serve.

PER SERVING: 338 calories, 28g protein, 20g fat, 11g carbohydrates, 3g fiber

Make it plant-based:
Replace the shrimp with edamame or adzuki beans. Check the label of your kimchi to make sure it's plant-based.

Chilled Cucumber-Avocado Soup with Spicy Shrimp

This refreshing cold soup has mint but isn't minty and has hot sauce but isn't spicy; it is just creamy and bright and full of flavor. The chili powder on the shrimp balances the bright soup and makes it hearty enough for a light summer meal. Tip: If you don't add water to thin it, you can use the avocado mixture as a dip.

PREP: 15 minutes
COOK: 10 minutes
SERVES: 4

1 pound medium shrimp, peeled and deveined, patted dry
1 tablespoon extra-virgin olive oil, plus more for drizzling
½ teaspoon chili powder
Fine sea salt and freshly ground black pepper
2 medium ripe avocados, halved and pitted
1 medium English cucumber, ends trimmed and chopped (about 2 cups)
¼ cup full-fat yogurt
1 teaspoon lime zest
¼ cup lime juice
2 tablespoons chopped fresh mint

1 teaspoon coconut aminos
1 teaspoon hot sauce, plus more for garnish
½ to 1 teaspoon raw honey (optional)

1. Preheat the oven to 400°F; line a large, rimmed baking sheet with parchment paper.
2. In a medium bowl, combine the shrimp, olive oil, and chili powder; toss. Season with salt and pepper. Spread on the baking sheet in a single layer and bake for 8 to 10 minutes, until just cooked through and pink. Transfer to a cutting board.
3. Squeeze the avocado flesh out of the skins into a blender. Add the cucumber, yogurt, lime zest and juice, mint, coconut aminos, and honey if using; blend until smooth. Thin with water, if needed, to reach the desired consistency. Taste and season with salt and pepper. (This will yield about 2¼ cups.)
4. Coarsely chop the shrimp. Divide the soup among 4 shallow bowls. Top with the shrimp. Drizzle with oil, sprinkle with parsley and/or add a few shakes of hot sauce, if desired, and serve.

PER SERVING: 373 calories, 32g protein, 24g fat, 7g carbohydrates, 4g fiber

Make it plant-based:
Omit the shrimp.

Shrimp Louie Salad–Stuffed Avocado

Creamy, tangy shrimp Louie is a classic, for good reason—it's easy to make and so delicious. Here we spoon it on top of avocado halves for a hearty lunch. With plenty of protein and healthy fats, it will leave you satisfied for hours. Have it on a toasted cauliflower round instead if avocado isn't your thing or isn't readily available.

PREP: 25 minutes
COOK: 10 minutes
SERVES: 4

1½ pounds medium shrimp, peeled and deveined

1 tablespoon extra-virgin olive oil

Fine sea salt and freshly grated black pepper

⅓ cup avocado oil mayonnaise

¼ cup ketchup (preferably unsweetened, such as Primal Kitchen)

¼ cup finely minced cornichons or sour pickle (8 to 10 cornichons)

½ teaspoon coconut aminos

¼ teaspoon hot sauce (optional)

2 ribs celery, minced (about ⅓ cup)

½ small red bell pepper, seeded and minced (about ½ cup)

2 teaspoons minced fresh dill

2 ripe avocados, halved, pitted, and peeled

1. Preheat the oven to 400°F. Line a large baking sheet with parchment paper.
2. Pat the shrimp dry thoroughly. Toss with the olive oil to coat; sprinkle with salt and pepper. Spread the shrimp in a single layer on the baking sheet and roast for 8 to 10 minutes, until just cooked through and pink. Transfer to a cutting board to cool.
3. In a small bowl, whisk together the mayonnaise, ketchup, pickle, coconut aminos, and hot sauce if using. Taste and season with salt and pepper. (This will yield about ¾ cup.)
4. When the shrimp is cool, coarsely chop. Place in a large bowl; add the celery and bell pepper. Add 4 to 5 tablespoons of the dressing and the dill; fold together. Fold in more dressing, if desired. Taste and season with salt and pepper. (This will yield about 3½ cups.)
5. Place an avocado half on each of 4 plates. Season lightly with salt and pepper. Spoon shrimp salad onto the avocado halves, piling in the center. Serve, passing additional dressing on the side.

PER SERVING: 498 calories, 42g protein, 33g fat, 13g carbohydrates, 6g fiber

Mussels in Spicy Tomato-Chorizo Broth

Mussels feel fancy, but they're actually incredibly fast and easy to cook, and very economical, too. Chorizo gives this dish depth and smokiness, but if you prefer to leave it out, stir in ½ teaspoon of smoked paprika when you add the garlic. Use a pot large enough so the mussels have some space and aren't too stacked on top of each other; that will take longer. Toss any that haven't opened after 10 minutes; they're unsafe to eat.

PREP: 15 minutes
COOK: 20 minutes
SERVES: 4

> 1 tablespoon avocado oil
> 3 ounces Spanish-style chorizo, chopped
> 1 small yellow onion, chopped (about 1 cup)
> Fine sea salt and freshly ground black pepper
> 3 garlic cloves, chopped (1 tablespoon)
> ½ teaspoon hot paprika
> ¼ teaspoon crushed red pepper flakes
> 1 14-ounce can fire-roasted diced tomatoes
> ½ cup dry white wine
> 3 sprigs fresh thyme
> 4 pounds mussels, scrubbed and debearded
> Toasted grain-free bread, mashed cauliflower or potatoes, cooked polenta, or
>   cooked zoodles, for serving (optional)

1. Warm the avocado oil in a Dutch oven or large pot over medium heat. Add the chorizo; cook for 2 to 3 minutes, stirring, until heated through. Add the onion, sprinkle with salt, and cook for 4 to 5 minutes, stirring, until tender. Add the garlic; sauté for 1 minute, until fragrant. Stir in the paprika and red pepper flakes.

2. Stir in the tomatoes and wine; stir to pull up any browned bits from the bottom of the pan. Stir in the thyme sprigs. Add the mussels and

stir to coat them with the sauce. Cover and cook for 8 to 10 minutes, stirring once or twice, until the mussels have opened. (Discard any mussels that haven't opened after 10 minutes.)

3. Serve hot with toasted bread, zoodles, mashed cauliflower, or other accompaniments, if desired.

PER SERVING: 335 calories, 35g protein, 11g fat, 18g carbohydrates, 2g fiber

Tuna Puttanesca–Stuffed Tomatoes

Puttanesca brings together tangy, briny favorites like capers, olives, and anchovies. Instead of serving this over the traditional pasta, here we add oil-packed tuna and stuff it into tomatoes for a delicious, no-cook, no-fuss meal that's loaded with flavor along with protein and healthy fats.

PREP: 20 minutes
SERVES: 4

4 medium tomatoes
2 6.7-ounce jars tuna fillets packed in olive oil (such as Tonnino)
2 tablespoons drained capers, coarsely chopped
3 tinned anchovy fillets, minced
¼ cup chopped pitted oil-cured black olives, or kalamata
½ teaspoon dried oregano
⅛ teaspoon red pepper flakes (or more if you like heat)
Fine sea salt and freshly ground black pepper
Extra-virgin olive oil (optional)

1. Slice the tops off the tomatoes. Use a melon baller or spoon to scoop out the seeds and insides.
2. In a medium bowl, flake the tuna with a fork. Add the anchovies, olives, oregano, and red pepper flakes; stir with the fork until the mixture is well combined. Add the reserved oil from the jars of tuna. Taste and season with salt and pepper.

3. Season the inside of the tomatoes with salt and pepper. Spoon the tuna mixture into the tomatoes. Drizzle each with additional oil, if desired, and serve, or cover and refrigerate for up to 4 hours.

PER SERVING: 234 calories, 20g protein, 14g fat, 6g carbohydrates, 0g fiber

Salmon Cakes

Even avowed non-fish eaters can usually be talked into a patty. Canned salmon in this recipe saves you some time and money; look for skinless, boneless wild-caught salmon for the healthiest and easiest to work with. Pork panko is a flavorful, no-carb binder that also adds richness to these satisfying patties.

PREP: 15 minutes
COOK: 10 minutes
YIELD: 8 patties

> 2 14.75-ounce cans salmon, drained
> 1 cup pork panko (such as Bacon's Heir)
> ½ cup avocado oil mayonnaise
> 1 small shallot, minced (about ⅓ cup)
> 1½ tablespoons chopped fresh dill
> 1 teaspoon lemon zest
> 1 tablespoon lemon juice
> 2 teaspoons drained capers, minced
> 1 teaspoon Dijon mustard
> 2 large eggs, beaten
> Fine sea salt and freshly ground black pepper
> Avocado oil, for frying

1. In a large bowl, combine the salmon, panko, mayonnaise, shallot, dill, lemon zest and juice, capers, mustard, and eggs. Mix gently but thoroughly. Taste and season with salt and pepper. Portion into 8 pieces, then form into 3-inch-wide, ½-inch-thick patties.

2. Preheat the oven to 200°F; line a large, rimmed baking sheet with a cooling rack. Place in the oven.

3. Warm 1 inch of avocado oil in a large nonstick skillet over medium heat. Add as many patties as will fit in a single layer with space between (do not overcrowd the skillet). Cook for 3 to 4 minutes, until golden on the bottom. Carefully flip and cook for 3 to 4 minutes longer, until golden on both sides and cooked through (cut a small slit on the center of one to check). Transfer to the baking sheet in the oven to keep warm. Repeat with more oil and patties until they're all cooked. Serve.

PER SERVING (1 PATTY): 379 calories, 42g protein, 23g fat, 3g carbohydrates, 0g fiber

NOTES:

There are endless ways to change the flavoring of these patties. Replace the shallots, citrus, capers, mustard, and spices with scallions, ginger, garlic, and a touch of toasted sesame oil for an Asian-inspired spin. Try parsley, cilantro, or tarragon instead of dill. Throw in some Old Bay seasoning or use chili powder and lime instead of lemon. Feel free to experiment and make them your own.

Also, try some of my sauces drizzled over these patties, such as the special sauce from the Upgraded Cheeseburgers (page 229), or the Tzatziki from the Lettuce-Wrapped Greek Lamb Meatballs with Tzatziki (page 234). Give the patties an Indian spin with curry powder and lime, and serve them with jarred chutney, or mix wasabi and honey into mayo for Asian salmon cakes. Or whisk jarred pesto into yogurt for a unique Mediterranean sauce.

Thai Fish and Vegetable Curry

Why order takeout when you can make a rich, flavorful curry at home? With plenty of vegetables, aromatics, and luscious coconut milk, this dish is perfect for a chilly night. You poach the fish right in the sauce, so it's simple, too. Cook up some cauli rice and you have a complete meal in one bowl.

PREP: 20 minutes
COOK: 25 minutes
SERVES: 4

> 2 tablespoons avocado oil
>
> 4 ounces shiitake mushrooms, sliced (about 2½ cups)
>
> Fine sea salt
>
> 1 small head broccoli, stem peeled and sliced, florets cut into bite-size pieces (about 2 cups)
>
> 1 medium bell pepper (red, yellow, or orange), seeded and chopped (1 cup)
>
> 4 scallions, white and light green parts sliced on a diagonal (about ⅓ cup)
>
> 2 tablespoons minced fresh ginger
>
> 3 garlic cloves, minced (1 tablespoon)
>
> 1 tablespoon jarred lemongrass, minced
>
> 2 tablespoons red curry paste
>
> 1 13.5-ounce can full-fat coconut milk
>
> 2 tablespoons lime juice
>
> 2 tablespoons fish sauce
>
> 1 pound cod or haddock, patted dry, cut into 2-inch pieces
>
> Freshly ground black pepper
>
> Fresh cilantro leaves, for garnish (optional)

1. Warm 1 tablespoon of the avocado oil in a large saucepan over medium-high heat. Add the mushrooms, season with salt, and cook for 6 to 8 minutes, stirring occasionally, until the mushrooms release their water and turn golden. Add the remaining 1 tablespoon oil and the broccoli, season lightly with salt, and cook for 1 to 2 minutes, stirring, until bright green. Add the bell peppers and scallions, sprinkle with salt, and cook for about 1 minute, stirring, until they are beginning to get tender.

2. Add the ginger and garlic; sauté for about 1 minute, until fragrant. Whisk in the lemongrass, curry paste, coconut milk, lime juice, and

fish sauce. Bring to a simmer. Reduce the heat to medium-low. Tuck
the fish pieces into the liquid, cover, and simmer for 5 to 7 minutes,
until the fish is cooked through. Taste and season with salt and
pepper.

3. Portion rice into 4 bowls, if using. Spoon the curry over each.
    Garnish with cilantro, if desired, and serve.

PER SERVING: 395 calories, 20g protein, 27g fat, 14g carbohydrates,
3g fiber

NOTE:
If you like your curry thicker, dissolve ½ teaspoon arrowroot in
½ teaspoon water and stir it in before adding the fish.

Make it plant-based:
Omit the fish.

Sheet-Pan Salmon and Broccoli with Lemon-Pepper Butter

A sheet-pan meal makes cleanup a breeze, perfect for busy weeknights.
You can make the lemon-pepper butter a few days ahead, so prep it on
Sunday and your weeknight self will thank you. If you have any left
over, enjoy it on scrambled eggs, steak, or steamed vegetables. Swap
the broccoli for another vegetable (or mix of vegetables), if you like.

PREP: 20 minutes
COOK: 20 minutes
SERVES: 4

Compound Butter:
  2 ounces unsalted butter, softened
  ½ teaspoon lemon zest
  1 teaspoon lemon juice
  ¼ teaspoon coarsely ground black pepper
  Fine sea salt

Salmon and Broccoli:
> *3 small or 1 large head broccoli, stems peeled and sliced, florets cut into*
> *bite-size pieces (about 7 cups)*
> *3 tablespoons extra-virgin olive oil*
> *4 4- to 6-ounce salmon fillets*

1. Preheat the oven to 425°F; place a large, rimmed baking sheet in the oven as it preheats.
2. Make the butter: In a small bowl, combine the butter, lemon zest and juice, pepper, and a generous pinch of salt. Mash together with a fork until incorporated. (You can make the butter up to 2 days ahead. Roll into a cylinder, wrap in plastic, and keep refrigerated. Cut into slices when you're ready to serve.)
3. Make the salmon and broccoli: Place the broccoli in a medium-sized salad bowl; add 2 tablespoons of the olive oil, season with salt, and toss. Spread on the baking sheet in a single layer and roast for 10 minutes. Stir and roast for 5 minutes longer. Meanwhile, prepare the salmon: Pat the fish dry and rub with the remaining 1 tablespoon oil. Season all over with salt.
4. Remove the hot baking sheet from the oven. Stir the broccoli and push to both sides of the baking sheet. Place the salmon skin-side down on the baking sheet. Return to the oven and roast for 4 to 8 minutes for medium-rare, until the salmon is cooked through to the desired doneness (cut into the thickest part of one piece to check the doneness; plan to roast for about 4 to 6 minutes per ½ inch of thickness).
5. Divide the broccoli among 4 plates. Place a piece of salmon on each. Top each with a dollop of the butter and serve.

PER SERVING: 559 calories, 43g protein, 38g fat, 11g carbohydrates, 4g fiber

NOTE:
If you like your broccoli more caramelized, roast it for 5 minutes longer before adding the salmon.

Chipotle-Bacon Scallops

There are two secrets to beautifully seared scallops: patting them as dry as you can, and getting your pan screaming hot. Do both of those things, and you'll be rewarded with restaurant-quality scallops without leaving your house. The side muscle is a little piece of hard flesh on the side of the scallop; simply pull it off with your fingers or trim it off with a paring knife.

PREP: 5 minutes
COOK: 15 minutes
SERVES: 4

> *2 slices bacon*
> *1 pound sea scallops, patted dry and side muscle removed*
> *½ teaspoon chipotle chili powder*
> *Fine sea salt and freshly ground black pepper*
> *1 tablespoon chopped fresh cilantro*
> *1 tablespoon lime juice*
> *Mixed greens, jarred salsa, sliced avocado, and lime wedges, for serving (optional)*

1. Place the bacon in a large, unheated skillet. Place over medium-low heat and cook for 6 to 8 minutes, until the bacon is golden and crisp and the fat has rendered. Transfer the bacon to a cutting board.
2. Raise the heat under the skillet to medium-high. Dust the scallops with the chili powder and sprinkle with salt and pepper. Place them in the skillet and cook for 2 to 3 minutes, until they're seared on one side. Turn and cook for 1 to 2 minutes longer, until seared on the other side (do not overcook). Don't overcrowd the skillet; work in batches if needed.
3. Chop or crumble the bacon. Divide the scallops among 4 plates. Sprinkle with the bacon, cilantro, and lime juice. Serve with greens, salsa, avocado, and lime wedges, if desired.

PER SERVING: 120 calories, 18g protein, 3g fat, 3g carbohydrates, 0g fiber

Fish and Vegetables en Papillote

Shhh—don't tell anyone how easy this meal is. It looks and sounds so impressive, but actually it's just a really simple assembly. The fish and vegetables steam inside the parchment paper, so there's no fish smell, and it's nearly impossible to mess it up. If you feel intimidated by cooking fish, start here.

PREP: 20 minutes
COOK: 20 minutes
SERVES: 4

> 1 small lemon, scrubbed, cut into 8 thin slices
> 4 4- to 6-ounce halibut or cod fillets, patted dry
> Fine sea salt and freshly ground black pepper
> 4 tablespoons jarred pesto
> 2 medium carrots, shredded (about 1 cup)
> 1 small zucchini, shredded (about 1 cup)
> 2 tablespoons minced pitted mild green or black olives (such as Castelvetrano)
> 4 tablespoons extra-virgin olive oil

1. Preheat the oven to 450°F. Fold 4 14-by-12-inch sheets of parchment paper in half; cut a large heart shape out of each.
2. Place 2 lemon slices on the right side of the fold on one parchment heart; repeat with remaining lemon slices and parchment hearts. Season the fish with salt and pepper; place one piece on top of the lemon slices on each piece of parchment paper. Spread 1 tablespoon pesto over each fish fillet. Top each with one-fourth of the carrots, zucchini, and olives. Drizzle each with 1 tablespoon olive oil. Season with salt and pepper.
3. Starting at the top of the curve of the heart, tightly fold the edge of the paper over. Continue folding tightly, overlapping the folds to

form a seal. Fold all the way down to the bottom, so the packet is sealed. Repeat with the remaining packets. Place the packets on a large, rimmed baking sheet.

4. Bake for 15 to 20 minutes (depending on the thickness of the fish), until the packets are puffed and lightly browned. Carefully open the packets (keep your fingers away from where the steam escapes so you don't get burned). Transfer the fish and vegetables to 4 plates and serve.

PER SERVING: 414 calories, 36g protein, 28g fat, 6g carbohydrates, 1g fiber

NOTE:

You can change up the style of this dish really easily. Omit the pesto and olives, add sliced ginger and garlic, and swap toasted sesame oil for olive oil and you have an Asian version. Use thinly sliced bell peppers, canned black olives, garlic, and chili powder for a Mexican-style variation. Change it up to suit your taste and what you have on hand.

CHICKEN RECIPES

Creamy Pesto Chicken-Spinach Casserole

Who doesn't love a creamy, comforting casserole? This one is secretly healthy, with plenty of protein and healthy fats, and very low on starch thanks to cauliflower rice. You can use precooked chicken in here if you happen to have leftovers. (Pro tip: This is also great for leftover holiday turkey.) Using thawed frozen cauliflower rice is a time-saver. Don't worry about the volume of spinach; it will seem like a ton, but it cooks down to just the right amount.

PREP: 30 minutes
COOK: 1 hour
SERVES: 8

1½ *pounds skinless, boneless chicken thighs, patted dry*
2 *tablespoons avocado oil*
Fine sea salt and freshly ground black pepper
2 *shallots, sliced*
10 *ounces baby spinach, chopped*
6 *garlic cloves, minced (2 tablespoons)*
¾ *cup avocado oil mayonnaise*
¾ *cup canned full-fat coconut milk*
1 *tablespoon lemon juice*
3 *tablespoons jarred pesto*
2 *large eggs, beaten*
12 *ounces frozen cauliflower rice, thawed*
Olive oil cooking spray
¼ *cup sliced almonds*

1. Preheat the oven to 425°F; place a large, rimmed baking sheet in the oven as it preheats.
2. Rub the chicken with 1 tablespoon of the avocado oil; season with salt and pepper. Carefully remove the hot sheet pan from the oven. Place the chicken on the pan and roast for 20 to 25 minutes, until cooked through, turning once halfway through. Transfer to a cutting board to cool slightly. Reduce the oven temperature to 375°F.
3. While the chicken is roasting, warm the remaining 1 tablespoon oil in a large skillet over medium heat. Add the shallots, sprinkle with salt, and cook for about 4 minutes, stirring, until tender. Add the spinach a handful at a time, tossing in the garlic as you go. Season with salt and pepper and cook for about 5 minutes, stirring, until the spinach wilts. Remove from the heat.
4. In a large bowl, whisk together the mayonnaise, coconut milk, lemon juice, pesto, and eggs. Fold in the cauliflower rice. When the chicken is cool enough to handle, shred or chop it and add it to the bowl, along with the spinach mixture. Fold until well combined.
5. Mist a 9-by-13-inch baking dish with cooking spray. Spread the rice mixture evenly in the baking dish. Sprinkle with the almonds; mist

the top with cooking spray. Bake for 25 to 30 minutes, until the casserole is warmed through and lightly bubbling on the edges. Let cool for 5 minutes before serving.

PER SERVING: 486 calories, 19g protein, 44g fat, 5g carbohydrates, 2g fiber

Chicken Sausage with Sauerkraut and Apple

Here's a quick skillet meal that utilizes precooked chicken sausage and pre-shredded coleslaw mix—great shortcuts for busy weeknights. It's loaded with flavor from the sauerkraut and apple, it's got plenty of satisfying protein, and it only requires one pan, so cleanup is a breeze.

PREP: 15 minutes
COOK: 20 minutes
SERVES: 4

> 2 tablespoons avocado oil
> 6 3-ounce links chicken sausage (preferably garlic flavored), sliced on a
> diagonal
> 1 medium onion, chopped (about 1½ cups)
> Fine sea salt and freshly ground black pepper
> 1 12-ounce package coleslaw mix (shredded cabbage and carrots)
> ¼ cup chicken bone broth
> 1 small tart apple (such as Granny Smith), finely chopped
> ½ cup drained fermented sauerkraut, chopped

1. Warm 1 tablespoon of the avocado oil in a large skillet over medium heat. Add the sausage and cook for 6 to 8 minutes, stirring occasionally, until golden. Transfer to a bowl; cover to keep warm.
2. Warm the remaining 1 tablespoon oil in the same skillet. Add the onion, sprinkle with salt, and cook for 3 to 5 minutes, stirring occasionally, until very tender. Add the coleslaw mix, season with

salt and pepper, and cook for 1 to 2 minutes, stirring, until tender and bright green. Pour in the broth; stir up any browned bits from the bottom of the skillet and cook for about 1 minute, until the liquid has mostly evaporated.

3. Stir in the apple; sauté for 1 minute. Add the sausage back to the skillet, along with any liquid that has collected in the bowl. Add the sauerkraut. Cook for about 1 minute, stirring, to just warm the sauerkraut and combine all of the ingredients. Serve.

PER SERVING: 397 calories, 24g protein, 20g fat, 30g carbohydrates, 7g fiber

Sheet-Pan Roasted Chicken Sausage and Vegetables

Think of this as a formula rather than a recipe. Of course you can follow it as written, but it also has endless possibilities for variation. Swap vegetables, especially in season (use asparagus in the spring, or delicata squash in the fall), change up the sausage (add a spicy one if you like heat), add different seasonings (Italian seasoning, zaatar, curry). There are a zillion ways to make this your own. Generally, 10 cups of chopped vegetables and 1½ pounds of sausage is a good ratio—after that, it's up to you.

PREP: 20 minutes
COOK: 40 minutes
SERVES: 4

2 medium heads broccoli, stems peeled and sliced, florets cut into bite-size
     pieces (about 5 cups)
4 medium carrots, sliced on a diagonal (about 2 cups)
1 medium red onion, sliced (about 2 cups)
1 bunch radishes (about 12), halved (quartered if large; about 1 cup)
6 whole garlic cloves, quartered lengthwise
3 tablespoons extra-virgin olive oil

Fine sea salt and freshly ground black pepper

8 3-ounce chicken sausage links (such as Aidells Artichoke & Garlic), sliced on a diagonal

2 teaspoons red wine, white wine, or sherry vinegar

1. Preheat the oven to 400°F; place 2 large, rimmed baking sheets in the oven as it preheats.
2. In a large bowl, combine the broccoli, carrots, red onion, radishes, and garlic. Add the olive oil; toss. Season with salt and pepper. Carefully remove the baking sheets from the oven and divide the vegetables between the baking sheets. Roast for 20 minutes, or until the vegetables are tender and beginning to caramelize.
3. Stir the vegetables, move them to one side of each baking sheet, and divide the sausage between the baking sheets. Roast for 15 to 20 minutes longer, stirring once, until the vegetables are very tender and caramelized and the sausage is warmed through.
4. Sprinkle with the wine; stir. (This will yield about 9 cups.) Divide among 4 bowls and serve.

PER SERVING: 399 calories, 26g protein, 23g fat, 24g carbohydrates, 7g fiber

New-Fashioned Chicken Waldorf Salad

The classic Waldorf salad, a mix of celery, apple, and mayo, dates back to the very first charity ball at the Waldorf Hotel in 1893, according to Food Network. Here's an update, with chicken and fennel, and added zing in the dressing thanks to lemon, parsley, and a touch of honey. It's super flavorful, with sweet, savory, and tangy elements. Plus, it's a fantastic way to use up leftover chicken when you have it.

PREP: 20 minutes
COOK: 10 minutes
SERVES: 4

Dressing:

½ cup full-fat Greek yogurt

3 tablespoons avocado oil mayonnaise

1 tablespoon minced fresh flat-leaf parsley

1 teaspoon lemon zest

2 teaspoons lemon juice

1 teaspoon raw honey

Fine sea salt and freshly ground black pepper

Salad:

½ cup chopped walnuts

8 ounces chopped cooked skinless, boneless chicken (leftovers, or from a
rotisserie bird; about 2½ cups)

1 large green apple, cored, chopped (1¾ cups)

½ medium fennel bulb, trimmed, halved, cored, and chopped (1 cup)

2 ribs celery, sliced on a diagonal (⅓ cup)

½ cup halved seedless red grapes

1 head Bibb or Boston lettuce

1. Make the dressing: In a large bowl, whisk together the yogurt,
   mayonnaise, parsley, lemon zest and juice, and honey. Taste and
   season with salt and pepper. (This will yield about ½ cup. You can
   make the dressing up to 1 day ahead; cover and refrigerate. Whisk
   before using.)
2. Make the salad: Preheat the oven to 350°F. Spread the walnuts on a
   rimmed baking sheet. Bake for 8 to 10 minutes, until toasted and
   fragrant, shaking the pan once during baking time. Transfer to a
   small bowl to cool.
3. Add the chicken, apple, fennel, celery, and grapes to the bowl with
   the dressing; gently fold together until all of the ingredients are
   incorporated. (This will yield about 5 cups.) Divide the lettuce
   among 4 shallow bowls. Top each with one-fourth of the chicken
   mixture, sprinkle with walnuts, and serve.

PER SERVING: 289 calories, 19g protein, 16g fat, 20g carbohydrates, 5g fiber

Make it plant-based:
Instead of chicken, stir in drained canned chickpeas. For the dressing, use plant-based yogurt and mayo, and sweeten with maple syrup instead of honey.

Better-Than-Grandma's Roast Chicken and Vegetables

There's something so comforting about a roast chicken—and the aroma as it's cooking is magical. The secret to a well-seasoned, juicy, flavor-packed bird is a dry brine. Salt the bird very well, put it on a plate, and let it sit in the fridge uncovered overnight. It's simple to do and you won't believe the difference. Swap the vegetables for others, if you prefer: baby potatoes, celery root, carrots, onion—you can't go wrong.

PREP: 25 minutes
CHILL: 8 hours
COOK: 1 hour 30 minutes
SERVES: 4

> 1 4- to 5-pound whole chicken
> Fine sea salt
> 5 sprigs fresh thyme
> 3 sprigs fresh rosemary
> 6 garlic cloves
> 1 lemon, quartered
> 1 medium sweet potato, scrubbed and dried, cut into ½-inch cubes
> 3 large shallots, cut into ½-inch-thick slices
> 1 medium bulb fennel, trimmed, cut into wedges
> 4 tablespoons extra-virgin olive oil
> Freshly ground black pepper

1. Pat the chicken dry thoroughly; trim off excess fat. Season the chicken inside and out liberally with salt. Place on a plate and refrigerate uncovered for at least 8 hours.

2. Preheat the oven to 425°F. Stuff the cavity of the chicken with 2 sprigs thyme, 1 sprig rosemary, 2 garlic cloves, and as much of the lemon as you can fit. Tie the legs together with kitchen twine.

3. Combine the remaining 4 garlic cloves, the sweet potato, shallots, and fennel in a large roasting pan. Toss with 2 tablespoons of the olive oil; season with salt and pepper. Tuck the remaining 3 sprigs thyme and 2 sprigs rosemary into the vegetable mixture. Place a roasting rack on top.

4. Brush the chicken with the remaining 2 tablespoons olive oil; season with salt and pepper. Place the chicken in the roasting rack. Roast for 1 hour 15 minutes to 1 hour 30 minutes, until the chicken is golden and cooked through (an instant-read thermometer stuck into the thigh away from the bone should read 160°F). Stir the vegetables once or twice during the cooking time.

5. Transfer the chicken to a cutting board. Tent with foil and allow it to rest for 10 to 15 minutes. Place the vegetables on a platter (or divide among 4 plates), removing and discarding any herb sprigs. Carve the chicken and serve with the vegetables.

PER SERVING: 553 calories, 29g protein, 17g fat, 18g carbohydrates, 4g fiber

GOT LEFTOVERS?

If you have chicken left over, upgrade it the next day into an Asian-inspired salad. Pull the meat from the bones and chop. In a bowl, toss together chopped lettuce, shredded cabbage, shredded carrots, and sliced snap or snow peas. Add Mandarin orange segments, if you have them. Make a quick dressing: Whisk together 2 tablespoons avocado oil, 1 tablespoon unseasoned rice vinegar, 1 teaspoon white miso, 1 teaspoon coconut aminos, ½ teaspoon toasted sesame oil, and ¼ to ½ teaspoon mirin (or honey). Season with salt. Toss the dressing with the chicken and vegetables, sprinkle with sliced almonds or sesame seeds, and enjoy.

Sheet-Pan Chicken Fajitas

Family-pleasing fajitas are so easy—one marinade flavors both the meat and the vegetables. Spoon the cooked chicken into one bowl and the vegetables into another, put all the toppings on the table, and let everyone build their own. Swap shrimp for the chicken, if you like.

PREP: 20 minutes (plus 1–4 hours of marinating time)
COOK: 35 minutes
SERVES: 4

Fajitas:

¼ cup avocado oil

1 tablespoon coconut aminos

1 tablespoon lime juice

2 teaspoons chili powder

1 teaspoon garlic powder

1 teaspoon dried oregano

½ teaspoon ground cumin

½ teaspoon smoked paprika

Fine sea salt and freshly ground black pepper

1½ pounds skinless, boneless chicken thighs, patted dry, trimmed, and cut into 1- to 2-inch pieces

1 small red onion, cut into ¼-inch slices

3 medium bell peppers (any color), seeded, cut into ½-inch slices

1 small jalapeño, seeds removed, thinly sliced crosswise

Warmed grain-free tortillas or cooked cauliflower rice, chopped avocado, cilantro, and/or other toppings, for serving (optional)

Crema:

⅓ cup sour cream

2 tablespoons lime juice

½ teaspoon coconut aminos

¼ teaspoon raw honey

⅛ teaspoon chili powder, or more to taste
Fine sea salt and freshly ground black pepper

1. Make the fajitas: In a large bowl, whisk together the avocado oil,
    coconut aminos, lime juice, chili powder, garlic powder, oregano,
    cumin, and smoked paprika. Whisk in ½ teaspoon salt and
    ¼ teaspoon pepper. Transfer half to a medium bowl. Place the
    chicken in the medium bowl. Place the onion, bell peppers, and
    jalapeño in the large bowl with the remaining marinade. Stir both
    until the ingredients are covered with the marinade. Cover and
    refrigerate for at least 1 hour or up to 4 hours.
2. Make the crema: In a small bowl, whisk together the sour cream,
    lime juice, coconut aminos, honey, and chili powder. Taste and
    season with salt and pepper. Whisk in more chili powder, if desired.
    Cover and refrigerate.
3. Preheat the oven to 425°F; place 2 baking sheets in the oven as it
    preheats.
4. Drain the vegetables; sprinkle with salt and pepper. Spread on one of
    the hot baking sheets and roast for 10 minutes. Spread the chicken
    on the other baking sheet and season with salt and pepper. Roast for
    20 to 25 minutes, until cooked through, flipping once (stir the
    vegetables when you flip the chicken; remove them if they're
    browning too much).
5. Serve the vegetables and chicken with the crema and tortillas or
    cauliflower rice, and any toppings, if desired.

PER SERVING: 504 calories, 26g protein, 41g fat, 14g carbohydrates,
3g fiber

Make it plant-based:
Omit the chicken and serve the roasted vegetables with pinto or black
beans. Use a plant-based plain yogurt instead of the sour cream in the
crema.

EGG RECIPES

Fennel, Shallot, and Goat Cheese Frittata

Frittatas are such a gift. They're easy to make, versatile, inexpensive, delicious hot or cold, and great any time of day. A frittata is also a great place to use up odds and ends in the fridge, like leftover vegetables and fresh herbs that are on their way out. Try a different type of cheese (or no cheese). It's hard to mess up, so have fun with it.

PREP: 10 minutes
COOK: 25 minutes
SERVES: 4

1 tablespoon unsalted butter
1 tablespoon avocado oil
1 small bulb fennel, trimmed, quartered, cored, and sliced (about 1½ cups)
2 shallots, chopped (about 1 cup)
Fine sea salt and freshly ground black pepper
2 garlic cloves, minced (2 teaspoons)
1 teaspoon fresh thyme leaves
2 tablespoons finely chopped pitted kalamata olives
10 large eggs
2 ounces soft goat cheese, crumbled

1. Preheat the oven to 400°F.
2. Warm a cast-iron skillet over medium heat. Melt the butter with the avocado oil. Add the fennel and shallots, sprinkle with salt and pepper, and cook for 5 to 7 minutes, stirring often, until the vegetables are tender and beginning to lightly caramelize. Add the garlic and thyme; sauté for 1 minute. Sprinkle the olives all over.
3. Beat the eggs with ½ teaspoon salt and ¼ teaspoon pepper. Pour into the skillet over the vegetables. Sprinkle the goat cheese all over the top. Cook for 2 to 3 minutes, until the edges begin to set. Transfer

the skillet to the oven and cook for 10 to 12 minutes, until the center is just set. Let stand for 2 minutes before cutting into wedges and serving. Store the leftovers covered in the fridge.

PER SERVING: 352 calories, 18g protein, 26g fat, 10g carbohydrates, 2g fiber

Huevos Rancheros Salad

This version of a breakfast fave is made healthier with less starch and more vegetables, but it still packs all the flavors you love. Make the dressing a day in advance if you can; that gives the flavors time to develop, plus it will thicken in the fridge.

PREP: 30 minutes
COOK: 15 minutes
SERVES: 4

Dressing:
   4 tablespoons extra-virgin olive oil
   3 garlic cloves, minced (1 tablespoon)
   1 small jalapeño, seeded and minced (1 tablespoon)
   1 teaspoon lime zest
   2 tablespoons lime juice
   1 cup fresh cilantro leaves
   ½ cup full-fat plain yogurt
   1 teaspoon coconut aminos
   ½ teaspoon honey
   Fine sea salt and freshly grated black pepper

Salad:
   1 large head romaine, shredded (about 6 cups)
   1 cup chunky salsa
   1 ripe avocado, halved, pitted, and chopped
   6 radishes, trimmed, halved, and sliced
   2 tablespoons avocado oil

8 large eggs

Fine sea salt and freshly ground black pepper

½ cup lightly crushed grain-free tortilla chips (such as Siete Foods)
(optional)

1. Make the dressing: Combine 2 tablespoons of the olive oil, the garlic, and jalapeño in a small, unheated skillet. Place over low heat and cook until the mixture sizzles. Allow it to sizzle for 30 seconds, then transfer to a blender. Add the remaining 2 tablespoons olive oil, the lime zest and juice, cilantro, yogurt, coconut aminos, and honey; blend until smooth. Taste and season with salt and pepper. (This will yield 1 cup. You can make the dressing up to 1 day ahead; keep covered and refrigerated. The dressing will thicken in the fridge, so whisk before using.)

2. Make the salads: Preheat the oven to 250°F.

3. Divide the lettuce, salsa, avocado, and radishes among 4 shallow bowls. Warm 1 tablespoon of the avocado oil in a large nonstick skillet over medium-high heat. Crack 4 eggs into the skillet, season with salt and pepper, and fry for 2 to 5 minutes, to desired doneness, flipping once if you like. Transfer to a plate; keep warm in the oven. Repeat with the remaining 1 tablespoon avocado oil and 4 eggs.

4. Top each salad with 2 eggs. Drizzle each with 1 tablespoon dressing and sprinkle with crushed chips, if using. Serve immediately, passing additional dressing on the side.

PER SERVING: 331 calories, 13g protein, 26g fat, 11g carbohydrates, 4g fiber

Brussels Sprout Hash with Bacon and Eggs

When you shred Brussels sprouts, they cook more quickly. Plus, they're perfect when paired with bacon and eggs. Caramelized onion, vinegar, and broth softens the sprouts' harsh flavor. This is a perfect weekend brunch dish, but it's also a really fun, fuss-free dinner.

PREP: 15 minutes
COOK: 50 minutes
SERVES: 4

> *4 slices bacon*
> *1 small yellow onion, chopped (about 1¼ cups)*
> *Fine sea salt and freshly ground black pepper*
> *¼ teaspoon honey*
> *1 pound Brussels sprouts, trimmed and shredded (about 6½ cups)*
> *2 teaspoons cider vinegar*
> *¼ cup chicken bone broth*
> *2 tablespoons ghee*
> *8 large eggs*

1. Place the bacon in a large, unheated nonstick skillet. Place over medium-low heat and cook for 8 to 10 minutes, until golden and crisp, turning a few times. Transfer to a cutting board.
2. Add the onion to the skillet with the bacon fat. Season with salt and pepper and drizzle with the honey. Cook for 15 to 20 minutes, stirring occasionally, until the onion is very tender and caramelized (watch carefully at the end to prevent burning).
3. Raise the heat to medium-high. Add the sprouts, season with salt, and sauté for 1 to 2 minutes, until bright green. Add the vinegar; toss for 1 minute. Pour in the broth; cook for 1 to 2 minutes, stirring, until the liquid has evaporated. Spread the mixture in the skillet, press it down, and let it cook undisturbed for 30 seconds. Stir and repeat for 4 to 6 minutes longer, until the sprouts are very tender and lightly browned in spots. Transfer to a bowl; cover to keep warm. (This should yield about 4 cups.)
4. Melt 1 tablespoon of ghee in the same skillet. Crack 4 eggs into the skillet, season with salt and pepper, and cook for about 5 minutes, to desired doneness, flipping if desired. Transfer to a plate; cover to keep warm. Repeat with the remaining ghee and eggs. Chop or crumble the bacon.

5. Divide the Brussels sprout mixture among 4 shallow bowls; sprinkle with bacon. Top each with 2 eggs and serve.

PER SERVING: 306 calories, 18g protein, 21g fat, 11g carbohydrates, 4g fiber

Deviled Eggs 3 Ways

I love deviled eggs. They feel indulgent and festive, but they're such a healthy treat. And they're so versatile. Plus, sometimes it just feels really good to eat with your fingers. Here are three takes on deviled eggs—make them for a party, or just for yourself. They're full of protein and healthy fats, so they're truly satisfying.

. . . .

HOW TO HARD COOK EGGS

The easiest way to hard cook eggs is to steam them. Hard-cooked eggs are notoriously difficult to peel if the eggs are fresh; steaming them makes this process so much easier. The peels come right off. To steam eggs, fill a pan with about an inch of water, enough to come up to the bottom of your steamer basket. Place the steamer basket in the pot and bring the water to a boil. Turn off the heat and carefully add the eggs to the basket in a single layer (I use tongs for this to keep my hands away from the steam). Cover the pot and turn the heat to medium-high. Steam the eggs for 10 minutes if you like the yolks a little soft and bright orange, 12 to 14 minutes for fully hard-cooked. Transfer the eggs to a bowl of ice water to cool.

. . . .

Classic Deviled Eggs

PREP: 20 minutes
YIELD: 12 pieces

> 6 large hard-cooked eggs, peeled
> 3 tablespoons mayonnaise (preferably avocado oil or olive oil)
> ¾ teaspoon Dijon mustard
> ½ teaspoon raw cider vinegar

Dash of Worcestershire sauce
Fine sea salt and freshly ground black pepper
Paprika, for garnish (optional)

Cut the eggs in half lengthwise. Spoon the yolks into a medium bowl. Add the mayonnaise, mustard, vinegar, and Worcestershire sauce; mash with a fork to blend well. (Alternatively, if you have a small food processor, you can blend the filling ingredients until smooth.) Taste and season with salt and pepper. Spoon the filling into the egg whites, or spoon the filling into a resealable bag, seal, snip off a corner, and pipe the filling into the whites. Sprinkle with paprika, if desired. Serve, or cover and refrigerate for up to 2 days.

PER SERVING (2 PIECES): 126 calories, 6g protein, 11g fat, 0g carbohydrates, 0g fiber

"Miso Soup" Deviled Eggs

PREP: 25 minutes
YIELD: 12 pieces

2 tablespoons avocado oil
2 scallions, white and light green parts minced (about 1 tablespoon)
1 tablespoon minced fresh ginger
6 large hard-cooked eggs, peeled
2 teaspoons white miso
½ teaspoon mirin
¼ teaspoon toasted sesame oil (optional)
Fine sea salt
1 2-inch piece baked nori, snipped into pieces, for garnish (optional)

1. Combine the avocado oil, scallions, and ginger in a small, unheated skillet. Place over low heat and cook until the mixture begins to sizzle. Let it sizzle for 1 minute, then transfer to a bowl to cool.

2.   Cut the eggs in half lengthwise. Spoon the yolks into the bowl with the scallion mixture. Add the miso, mirin, and sesame oil if using. Mash with a fork to blend well. (Alternatively, if you have a small food processor, you can blend the filling ingredients until smooth.) Taste and season with salt, if needed.

3.   Spoon the filling into the egg whites, or spoon the filling into a resealable bag, seal, snip off a corner, and pipe the filling into the whites. Top each with a piece of nori, if desired, and serve, or cover and refrigerate for up to 2 days.

PER SERVING (2 PIECES): 127 calories, 6g protein, 10g fat, 1g carbohydrates, 0g fiber

NOTE:

The darker miso is, the saltier and more strongly flavored it is. White miso is best here, both for flavor and for aesthetics.

Beet-Horseradish Deviled Eggs

PREP: 20 minutes
YIELD: 12 pieces

> 6 large hard-cooked eggs, peeled
> 1 small steamed beet, chopped
> 2 tablespoons mayonnaise (preferably avocado oil or olive oil)
> 2 teaspoons drained jarred horseradish
> ¼ teaspoon raw cider vinegar
> Fine sea salt and freshly ground black pepper
> Snipped chives, for garnish (optional)

1.   Cut the eggs in half lengthwise. Spoon the yolks into the bowl of a small food processor. Add the beet, mayonnaise, horseradish, and vinegar; blend until smooth. Taste and season with salt and pepper.

2. Spoon the filling into the egg whites, or spoon the filling into a resealable bag, seal, snip off a corner, and pipe the filling into the whites. Top each with chives, if desired. Serve. (To make these in advance, keep the filling and whites in separate covered containers in the fridge for up to 1 day. Whisk to mix the filling before piping into the whites. If you fill them in advance, the beets will bleed onto the whites.)

PER SERVING (2 PIECES): 114 calories, 6g protein, 9g fat, 1g carbohydrates, 0g fiber

VEGETARIAN RECIPES

Cauliflower Gnocchi Caprese

If you love a caprese salad, you're in for a treat. This simple vegetarian meal combines all those flavors—basil, tomatoes, mozzarella—with filling cauliflower gnocchi. Roasting the gnocchi gives them better texture and is more hands off than cooking them in a skillet, so it's a win-win.

PREP: 10 minutes
COOK: 25 minutes
SERVES: 4

2 12-ounce packages frozen cauliflower gnocchi (such as Trader Joe's)
Olive oil cooking spray
¼ cup jarred pesto
2 tablespoons extra-virgin olive oil
2 cups halved cherry or grape tomatoes
1 cup halved fresh mozzarella balls
Fine sea salt and freshly ground black pepper

1. Preheat the oven to 425°F. Line a large baking sheet with parchment paper.

2. Spread the frozen gnocchi evenly on the baking sheet; mist with cooking spray. Roast for 20 to 25 minutes, until golden and cooked through, shaking the pan halfway through.

3. In a large bowl, whisk together the pesto and olive oil. When the gnocchi is finished, add it to the bowl and quickly toss to coat it with the pesto mixture. Add the tomatoes and cheese; gently toss. Taste and season with salt and pepper. Divide the mixture among 4 shallow bowls and serve.

PER SERVING: 380 calories, 10g protein, 23g fat, 31g carbohydrates, 9g fiber

Make it plant-based

Cut up a plant-based mozzarella, such as Miyoko's Kitchen, in place of the dairy cheese.

Dairy-Free Spaghetti Squash "Alfredo"

Noodles topped with a super-rich, creamy sauce is total comfort food—until afterward, when you're bloated from the dairy and crashing from the carbs. Here we swap spaghetti squash for the noodles and make a non-dairy alfredo with cashews, hemp hearts, and nutritional yeast—so you get all the comfort during and after.

PREP: 20 minutes
CHILL: 4 hours
COOK: 50 minutes
SERVES: 2 (or 4 as a side dish)

    1 cup raw cashews
    1 medium spaghetti squash (about 2½ pounds)
    3 tablespoons extra-virgin olive oil
    Fine sea salt and freshly ground black pepper
    2 garlic cloves, minced (2 teaspoons)
    1½ tablespoons lemon juice
    2½ tablespoons nutritional yeast

1 tablespoon hemp hearts
1 cup boiling water, plus ½ cup more as needed
1 tablespoon chopped fresh parsley
Crushed red pepper flakes (optional)

1. Place the cashews in a medium bowl. Cover with cool water. Cover and refrigerate for at least 4 hours, or overnight.

2. Preheat the oven to 400°F; line a large baking sheet with parchment paper.

3. Place the squash on a sturdy cutting board. Using a sharp chef's knife, slice off the rounded bottom part and stem end of the squash. Turn the squash so that it sits flat on the sliced-off bottom. Cut through the middle of the squash to halve it lengthwise. Using a tablespoon, scrape out the seeds.

4. Brush the inside of the squash with 1 tablespoon of the olive oil; season with salt and pepper. Place the squash cut-side down on the baking sheet. Roast for 40 to 50 minutes, until the squash is tender and easily pierced with a knife. Carefully turn it over and let it cool slightly.

5. Meanwhile, make the sauce. Combine the remaining 2 tablespoons oil and garlic in a small, unheated skillet. Place over low heat and cook until the mixture begins to sizzle. Allow it to sizzle for 1 minute, then transfer it to a blender. Drain the cashews. Rinse with cool water, shaking off excess, and transfer to the blender. Add the lemon juice, nutritional yeast, hemp hearts, and ½ cup boiling water; blend until well combined. Blend in more water, 1 to 2 tablespoons at a time, until the mixture is smooth and has reached sauce consistency. Taste and season with salt and pepper. (This will yield about 1½ cups.)

6. Using a fork, scrape the strands of spaghetti squash out of each half. (This will yield about 3½ cups.) If the squash is cool, sauté it quickly in a large skillet to rewarm. Toss with about half of the sauce, sprinkle with parsley and red pepper flakes (if desired), and serve.

PER SERVING: 676 calories, 18g protein, 50g fat, 46g carbohydrates, 9g fiber

NOTES:

Top this dish with leftover cooked vegetables. Add a protein, if you like, such as sliced cooked chicken or quick-sautéed shrimp.

Let the remaining sauce cool, then cover and refrigerate for up to 3 days. Use it with more squash, or with pasta.

Sesame Zoodles with Vegetables

Here's a vegetarian dish that's rich and luscious and works served hot, warm, or cold. Like the take-out noodle dish that inspired it, it has a creamy sauce with an almond butter base, rice vinegar, fresh ginger, and toasted sesame oil. We swap in zucchini noodles and add more vegetables to bump up the nutrition. Enjoy it this way or top it with your favorite protein.

PREP: 25 minutes
COOK: 15 minutes
SERVES: 4

> *3 tablespoons avocado oil*
> *3 scallions, white and light green parts, sliced on a diagonal, dark green parts sliced and reserved for garnish (optional)*
> *2 garlic cloves, minced (2 teaspoons)*
> *2 teaspoons minced fresh ginger*
> *½ cup creamy unsweetened almond butter*
> *3 tablespoons coconut aminos*
> *2 teaspoons unseasoned rice vinegar*
> *1 to 2 teaspoons sriracha (optional)*
> *1 tablespoon toasted sesame oil*
> *Fine sea salt and freshly ground black pepper*

1 medium red bell pepper, seeded, thinly sliced (about 1 cup)

1 cup snow peas, sliced

1 medium carrot, shredded (about ½ cup)

4 medium zucchini, summer squash, or a combination, spiralized (or about
*   12 to 14 ounces precut zucchini noodles)*

2 teaspoons sesame seeds, for garnish (optional)

1. Combine 2 tablespoons of the avocado oil, the scallions, garlic, and ginger in a medium skillet. Place over low heat and cook until the mixture begins to sizzle. Allow it to sizzle for 1 minute, then whisk in the almond butter, coconut aminos, rice vinegar, and sriracha if using. Cook, whisking, for 1 minute. Transfer to a large bowl, whisk in the sesame oil, and season with salt and pepper. Thin with hot water 1 tablespoon at a time, if needed, to reach a thick sauce consistency. (This will yield about 1 cup.)

2. Wipe out the skillet. Warm another ½ tablespoon oil in the skillet. Add the bell pepper and snow peas; season with salt and pepper. Cook for 3 to 4 minutes, stirring, until tender. Add the carrots; sauté for 1 to 2 minutes, until tender. Transfer to a large bowl and let cool.

3. Add the remaining ½ tablespoon oil to the skillet. Add the zucchini noodles, season with salt, and cook for 4 to 6 minutes, stirring, until just tender. Using tongs, lift the noodles out of the skillet; transfer to a colander to drain and cool.

4. Add the noodles to the bowl with the other vegetables. Add ¼ cup of the sauce; gently toss. Add more sauce, if desired, and toss. Using the tongs, toss until all of the ingredients are coated with the sauce. Taste and season with salt and pepper. (This will yield about 6 cups.) Divide among 4 bowls, sprinkle with sesame seeds and scallion greens, if desired, and serve at room temperature.

PER SERVING: 394 calories, 10g protein, 31g fat, 23g carbohydrates, 10g fiber

NOTES:

If you prefer this dish cold, instead of dividing it, cover the bowl and refrigerate to serve later.

If you prefer the sauce smoother, transfer the warmed scallion mixture to the bowl of a small food processor. Add the remaining ingredients and blend.

Leftover sauce makes a good salad dressing, dip for vegetables, or topping for grilled chicken.

ADDITIONAL RECIPES

Skillet Jambalaya with Cauliflower Rice

If you have a jar of Cajun seasoning in your pantry, you can skip making the spice mix and use that instead (you'll need 2½ tablespoons). In that case, check the label and see if your jar already has salt and pepper. If it does, don't add more as you go. Check the seasoning at the end to see if you need more salt and/or pepper.

PREP: 20 minutes
COOK: 35 minutes
SERVES: 4

Spice mix:

    1 teaspoon sweet paprika
    ½ teaspoon smoked paprika
    2 teaspoons garlic powder
    1½ teaspoons dried oregano
    1 teaspoon onion powder
    ½ teaspoon cayenne

Jambalaya:

    3 tablespoons avocado oil
    12 ounces medium shrimp, peeled and deveined

Fine sea salt and freshly ground black pepper

3 3-ounce links of andouille sausage (pork or chicken), sliced on a
diagonal

8 ounces skinless, boneless chicken thighs or breasts, cut into 1-inch pieces,
patted dry

1 12-ounce package frozen cauliflower rice

1 medium red bell pepper, seeded and chopped (1 cup)

2 ribs celery, chopped (¾ cup)

3 scallions, white and light green parts sliced (about ⅓ cup), dark green parts
reserved for garnish

1 15-ounce can fire-roasted diced tomatoes, drained with liquid reserved

¼ cup chicken bone broth

Hot sauce, for serving (optional)

1. Make the spice mix: In a small bowl, combine the sweet paprika, smoked paprika, garlic powder, oregano, onion powder, and cayenne.

2. Make the jambalaya: Warm 1 tablespoon of the avocado oil in a large skillet over medium-high heat. Add the shrimp, season with salt and pepper, and sprinkle with ½ teaspoon of the spice mix. Cook for 2 to 4 minutes, stirring, until the shrimp are just cooked through. Transfer to a large bowl.

3. Add the sausage to the skillet and cook for 5 to 7 minutes, stirring, until lightly browned. Transfer to the bowl with the shrimp. Warm another 1 tablespoon oil in the skillet. Add the chicken, season with salt and pepper, and sprinkle with ½ teaspoon of the spice mix. Cook for 6 to 8 minutes, stirring, until cooked through and beginning to turn golden in spots. Transfer to the bowl with the shrimp and sausage.

4. Add the cauliflower rice, season with salt and pepper, and cook for 4 to 5 minutes, stirring and pulling up browned bits from the bottom of the skillet, until the rice has thawed and warmed through. Add the bell pepper and celery, sprinkle with salt, and ½ teaspoon of the spice mix; cook for about 3 minutes, stirring, until tender. Add

the white and light green parts of the scallions and the remaining spice mix; sauté for 1 minute.

5. Stir in the tomatoes and broth. Add the proteins and any juices that have collected in the bowl. Reduce the heat to medium. Cook for 1 to 2 minutes, stirring, to rewarm the proteins and meld the flavors. If the mixture is dry, add the liquid from the canned tomatoes 1 tablespoon at a time until you reach the desired consistency. Taste and season with additional salt and pepper, if needed. (This will yield about 8 cups.)

6. Divide among 4 shallow bowls, sprinkle with hot sauce if desired, top with the dark scallion greens, and serve.

PER SERVING: 429 calories, 35g protein, 25g fat, 15g carbohydrates, 4g fiber

Make it plant-based

Leave out the chicken and shrimp. Use a plant-based sausage, and add some pinto beans.

Egg Roll Bowls

This fun family favorite lets you make a take-out favorite at home. It's easy to customize based on the protein you have on hand. Make sure that you have all your ingredients prepped before you start cooking; once the heat is on, it moves very quickly. Pass sriracha on the side if not everyone likes heat.

PREP: 20 minutes
COOK: 15 minutes
SERVES: 4

½ teaspoon arrowroot
¼ cup coconut aminos
1 tablespoon mirin
1½ teaspoons unseasoned rice vinegar (or cider vinegar)
1 teaspoon sriracha (optional)

2 tablespoons avocado oil

1½ pounds protein of choice (peeled and deveined shrimp, ground pork,
   ground turkey, chicken breast or thigh pieces)

Fine sea salt and freshly ground black pepper

6 scallions, white and light green parts sliced on a diagonal (¾ cup), dark
   green parts sliced and reserved for garnish (optional)

1 cup snow peas, sliced on a diagonal

3 garlic cloves, minced (1 tablespoon)

1 tablespoon minced fresh ginger

1 14- to 16-ounce bag coleslaw mix (shredded cabbage and carrots)

1 to 2 tablespoons toasted sesame oil

Additional sriracha and gluten-free hoisin, for serving (optional)

1. In a small cup, dissolve the arrowroot in ½ teaspoon water. In a cup,
   combine the coconut aminos, mirin, rice vinegar, and sriracha if
   using.

2. Warm 1 tablespoon of the avocado oil in a large skillet over medium-
   high heat. Add the protein, season with salt and pepper, and cook,
   stirring, until just cooked through (timing will depend on the type
   of protein). Remove to a plate and cover to keep warm. If there's
   excess liquid in the skillet, pour it off.

3. Warm the remaining 1 tablespoon oil in the skillet over medium-
   high heat. Add the white and light green parts of the scallions and
   the snow peas; sprinkle with salt and pepper and cook for 1 minute,
   stirring. Add the garlic and ginger; stir-fry for 1 minute, until
   fragrant. Add the coleslaw mix; season with salt and stir-fry for 1 to
   2 minutes, until tender.

4. Reduce the heat to medium. Add the protein back to the skillet along
   with any juices that collected on the plate. Whisk the coconut
   aminos mixture and pour it into the skillet, stirring to pull up
   any browned bits from the bottom of the skillet. Drizzle in the
   arrowroot mixture and cook about 1 minute longer, stirring, until
   the sauce reduces and thickens and coats all the ingredients in the
   skillet.

5. Remove from the heat and drizzle with 1 tablespoon of the sesame oil. Taste and season with additional salt, pepper, and/or sesame oil, if needed. Serve, garnishing with dark scallion greens, if desired. Pass the sriracha and hoisin on the side, if desired.

Make it plant-based

You can make this dish vegetarian by using defrosted shelled edamame or chopped baked tofu as the protein. There's no need to precook either, simply add either (or both) at the end when you would add any cooked protein and stir to warm through.

PER SERVING: 359 calories, 43g protein, 14g fat, 14g carbohydrates, 5g fiber

SIDES/TREATS

Grain-Free "Golden Milk" Banana Muffins

Banana muffins are a crowd pleaser, but if you want yours to stand out, try adding turmeric, ginger, and cinnamon, the spices in "golden milk," a healing warm drink from India. Turmeric's anti-inflammatory powers are well documented, cinnamon helps with blood-sugar regulation, and ginger has antioxidant properties. Plus, these muffins are so moist, luscious, and sweet, you won't believe they have no added sugar.

PREP: 15 minutes
BAKE: 25 minutes
YIELD: 12 muffins

> 2 cups blanched almond flour
> ¼ cup arrowroot
> 3 tablespoons collagen peptides
> 1 teaspoon baking soda
> 2 teaspoons ground cinnamon

1 teaspoon ground ginger

1 teaspoon ground turmeric

¼ teaspoon fine sea salt

3 medium ripe bananas

6 pitted dried dates

¼ cup extra-virgin olive oil

1 teaspoon vanilla extract

2 large eggs, beaten

1. Preheat the oven to 350°F; line a 12-cup muffin tin with paper liners.
2. In a large bowl, whisk together the almond flour, arrowroot, collagen, baking soda, cinnamon, ginger, turmeric, and salt.
3. In a blender or the bowl of a food processor, combine the bananas, dates, olive oil, and vanilla; blend until smooth. Add to the bowl with the flour mixture, along with the eggs. Fold together until all of the ingredients are well combined. Divide the batter among the muffin cups.
4. Bake for 20 to 25 minutes, until the muffins are golden and a toothpick inserted in the center of one comes out clean (cover with foil if the tops begin to brown too much). Let the muffins cool in the pan on a wire rack for 5 minutes, then transfer to the rack to cool completely. Store the leftovers covered in the fridge.

PER SERVING (1 MUFFIN): 226 calories, 16g fat, 7g protein, 16g carbohydrates, 3g fiber

Glazed Grain-Free Carrot Cake Muffins

Rich, spicy carrot cake, but in muffin form, minus the grains and refined sugar—what a treat. The coconut butter glaze is optional, but I recommend it; it makes the muffins so festive that they feel like cake, and adds a bit more healthy fat, too.

PREP: 15 minutes
BAKE: 25 minutes
YIELD: 12 muffins

> 1½ cups (168 grams) blanched almond flour
> ¼ cup (36 grams) arrowroot
> ¼ cup (40 grams) collagen peptides
> 2 teaspoons ground cinnamon
> 1 teaspoon ground ginger
> ¼ teaspoon ground nutmeg
> ½ teaspoon baking powder
> ¼ teaspoon baking soda
> ¼ teaspoon plus a pinch fine sea salt
> 3 large eggs, at room temperature
> ⅓ cup plus 2 tablespoons maple syrup
> 3 tablespoons extra-virgin olive oil
> 1¼ teaspoons vanilla extract
> 2 medium carrots, shredded (1 cup)
> ½ cup chopped walnuts or pecans
> ¼ cup unsweetened shredded coconut (optional)
> ¼ cup coconut butter

1. Preheat the oven to 350°F. Line a 12-cup muffin tin with paper liners.
2. In a large bowl, combine the almond flour, arrowroot, collagen, cinnamon, ginger, nutmeg, baking powder, baking soda, and ¼ teaspoon salt. In a separate medium bowl, whisk together the eggs, ⅓ cup of the maple syrup, the olive oil, and 1 teaspoon of the vanilla. Add the egg mixture to the flour mixture and stir until just incorporated. Fold in the walnuts and coconut if using.
3. Divide the batter among the muffin cups. Bake for 22 to 25 minutes, until golden and a toothpick inserted in the center of a muffin comes out clean. Transfer the pan to a wire rack; let the muffins cool for 5 minutes. Transfer the muffins to the rack to cool completely.

4. In a small bowl, whisk together the coconut butter and the
    remaining pinch of salt, the remaining 2 tablespoons maple syrup,
    and the remaining ¼ teaspoon vanilla. (If the coconut butter is very
    stiff, warm the ingredients in a small saucepan over low heat and
    whisk until well combined and softened.) When the muffins have
    cooled completely, spoon about 1 teaspoon glaze over each muffin;
    gently spread with the back of a spoon. Serve. Keep leftovers covered
    in the fridge.

PER SERVING (1 MUFFIN): 255 calories, 18g fat, 7g protein,
17g carbohydrates, 3g fiber

Chocolate Date-"Halvah" Bites

I love halvah, the Middle Eastern candy made from sesame seeds—but I
don't love all the sugar that's in it. These bites, made with tahini, get
their sweetness from dates instead (and a tiny touch of maple syrup).
They're nut free and make a perfect little sweet bite after a meal for
adults or kids.

PREP: 20 minutes
YIELD: About 22 pieces

> 1½ cups pitted dried dates
> ½ cup tahini
> ½ cup (48 grams) unsweetened cacao powder
> 1 tablespoon maple syrup
> 1 teaspoon vanilla extract
> ½ teaspoon instant coffee (optional)
> ¼ teaspoon fine sea salt

In the bowl of a food processor, pulse the dates until well chopped.
Add the tahini, cacao powder, maple syrup, vanilla, coffee if using,
and salt. Blend for 1 to 2 minutes, until smooth. Using a spoon or 1
tablespoon scoop, portion into 22 pieces. Roll each into a ball. Serve,

or cover and refrigerate (for up to 1 week) or freeze (for up to 2 months).

PER SERVING (1 PIECE): 80 calories, 3g fat, 2g protein, 12g carbohydrates, 2g fiber

NOTES:

Make sure you use soft dates for these, or they won't hold together. If your dates are hard, soak them in hot water for 10 to 15 minutes. Drain them and pat dry before proceeding.

You can roll these in toasted coconut, cacao nibs, sesame seeds, or chopped nuts, if you like.

Chocolate-Coconut Freezer Fudge

A healthier form of fudge? Yes, please. This one is made without refined sugar, and the coconut butter makes it so rich, you really can only eat a small portion. Plus, you keep it in the freezer, so you don't have to worry about using it up quickly to keep it from going bad. I like to make it in a mini muffin tin, but you can also freeze it in a baking dish, cut it into small squares, and freeze the pieces in a heavy resealable bag.

PREP: 20 minutes
FREEZE: 1 hour
YIELD: About 20 pieces

1 cup unsweetened coconut butter
2 tablespoons coconut oil
¼ cup (24 grams) unsweetened cacao powder
½ cup maple syrup
1 teaspoon vanilla extract
¼ teaspoon fine sea salt
Flaky sea salt (such as Maldon) (optional)

1. Line the cups of a 24-cup mini muffin tin with paper liners or line an 8-inch square baking dish with parchment paper or waxed paper.
2. In a large bowl set over a pan of simmering water, combine the coconut butter and coconut oil. Let stand until softened. Remove from the heat; whisk to combine.
3. Add the cacao, maple syrup, vanilla, and salt to the bowl. Whisk until smooth.
4. Divide the mixture among the muffin cups or spread in the baking dish. Sprinkle with flaky sea salt, if desired. Freeze until firm, at least 1 hour. Serve, or transfer to a freezer bag to keep frozen. (Once firm, you can cut the fudge into pieces if you have it in the baking dish, then transfer to a freezer bag.)

NOTE:

The fudge should be kept frozen and served out of the freezer. At room temperature it will begin to melt.

PER SERVING (1 PIECE): 110 calories, 1g protein, 9g fat, 9g carbohydrates, 2g fiber

Grain-Free Granola

Packaged granola has a health halo—but it's often loaded with sugar and made with grains and low-quality oil. Luckily, making it yourself is so simple, and then you control the ingredients. Think of this as a base recipe; change up the spices and the mix of nuts and seeds to suit your tastes. Homemade granola in a pretty jar makes a really lovely hostess gift, too.

PREP: 10 minutes
COOK: 45 minutes
YIELD: About 4 cups

> ¾ cup raw walnuts or pecans
> ½ cup raw pumpkin seeds

½ cup raw cashews

¾ cup raw sliced almonds

½ cup unsweetened shredded coconut

¼ cup hemp seeds

¼ cup extra-virgin olive oil

⅓ cup maple syrup

1 teaspoon vanilla extract

2 teaspoons cinnamon

½ teaspoon ground ginger

½ teaspoon fine sea salt

1. Preheat the oven to 300°F.
2. Coarsely chop the walnuts, pumpkin seeds, and cashews. Transfer to a large bowl, add the almonds, coconut, and hemp seeds. Toss.
3. Add the olive oil, maple syrup, vanilla, cinnamon, ginger, and salt; fold together until all of the ingredients are combined well. Spread evenly on a large, rimmed baking sheet.
4. Bake for 15 minutes. Stir, spread out evenly again, and continue to bake for 20 to 30 minutes longer, until very fragrant, golden, and toasted. Stir every 10 minutes. (Granola will crisp up as it cools.) Transfer to a large bowl to cool; stir a few times as it cools. Store the granola in an airtight container at room temperature for up to a week, in the refrigerator for up to 2 weeks, or in the freezer for up to 3 months.

PER SERVING (¼ CUP): 203 calories, 5g protein, 17g fat, 10g carbohydrates, 2g fiber

Sausage-Stuffed Mushrooms

This is one of my favorite appetizers—so I thought, why not have it all the time? It's really satisfying, it's loaded with protein, and you can make a big batch. Keep it covered in the fridge and just pop a few in the toaster oven to warm them up when you want a quick side dish.

PREP: 25 minutes
COOK: 30 minutes
YIELD: 20 pieces

> 20 button mushrooms, stems removed
> 3 tablespoons extra-virgin olive oil
> Fine sea salt and freshly ground black pepper
> 1 pound sweet or hot Italian sausage, casings removed
> 4 scallions, white and light green parts, minced (about ⅓ cup)
> 3 garlic cloves, minced (1 tablespoon)
> 4 tablespoons freshly grated Parmesan cheese
> ¼ cup (26 grams) blanched almond flour
> 1 tablespoon minced fresh parsley
> Olive oil cooking spray

1. Preheat the oven to 350°F. Line a large, rimmed baking sheet with parchment paper.
2. Place the mushrooms hollow-side up on the baking sheet. Brush the mushrooms with olive oil; season with salt and pepper.
3. Warm the remaining 1 tablespoon oil in a large skillet over medium heat. Add the sausage and cook for 8 to 10 minutes, stirring and breaking it up with a wooden spoon, until cooked through and lightly browned. Add the scallions and garlic; cook for about 2 minutes, stirring, until tender and fragrant. Stir in 3 tablespoons of the Parmesan, the almond flour, and the parsley; cook for 1 to 2 minutes, stirring, until well combined and warmed through. Taste and season with salt and pepper, if needed.
4. Fill each mushroom cap with stuffing. Bake for 10 to 12 minutes, until the mushrooms are cooked through and the filling is hot. Sprinkle each mushroom with the remaining 1 tablespoon Parmesan, mist with cooking spray, and bake for 3 minutes longer, until the cheese is golden.

PER SERVING (2 PIECES): 143 calories, 11g protein, 10g fat, 3g carbohydrates, 1g fiber

NOTE:

Medium to large mushrooms are best for this. Smaller ones are harder to fill. But if smaller ones are all that's available, buy 5 to 10 extra to be sure you use up all the filling.

Prosciutto-Wrapped Asparagus

For these simple, delicious bites, make sure you buy asparagus spears that are not too thin or too thick. The really thin, delicate ones get overdone in the time it takes the prosciutto to crisp, and the thick ones won't be done enough in that time. Medium spears work perfectly. There's no need to add salt; the prosciutto is salty enough, especially when roasted.

PREP: 10 minutes
COOK: 12 minutes
YIELD: 12 pieces

> *6 slices prosciutto*
> *12 medium-thick spears asparagus*
> *1 tablespoon extra-virgin olive oil*
> *Freshly ground black pepper*
> *1 teaspoon lemon juice (optional)*
> *Freshly grated Parmesan cheese (optional)*

1. Preheat the oven to 400°F. Line a large baking sheet with parchment paper.
2. Cut each slice of prosciutto in half lengthwise. Snap or cut off the woody ends of the asparagus. Place on the baking sheet and toss with olive oil. Starting just under the flowery tip of the asparagus, wrap a piece of prosciutto around each spear. Place back on the baking sheet. Season lightly with pepper.
3. Roast for 10 to 12 minutes, until the asparagus is tender and the prosciutto is crisp. Sprinkle with lemon juice and dip in Parmesan, if desired, and serve.

NOTE:

These are best eaten right out of the oven, when they're hot and crisp.
You can prepare the asparagus but not bake it; cover and refrigerate for
up to 2 days. Cook as needed in the oven or toaster oven.

PER SERVING (2 SPEARS): 96 calories, 9g protein, 7g fat,
1g carbohydrates, 1g fiber

Air Fryer Jicama "Fries" with Herbed Mayo

If you thought fries were off the menu, this one's for you. Instead of
potatoes, these are made from jicama (pronounced HICK-ah-mah), a
nutrient-rich tuber that's native to Mexico. Jicama is rich in prebiotic
fiber, which feeds the good bacteria in your gut, so it's a real health
booster. You can also enjoy it raw; it's crunchy and slightly sweet,
delicious with guac or other dips.

PREP: 25 minutes
COOK: 40 minutes
SERVES: 4

Herbed mayo:

1 tablespoon extra-virgin olive oil
1 clove garlic, minced (1 teaspoon)
½ cup avocado oil mayonnaise
1 teaspoon lemon zest
1 tablespoon lemon juice
3 tablespoons chopped fresh parsley
2 tablespoons chopped fresh dill
Fine sea salt and freshly ground black pepper

Jicama fries:

Fine sea salt
18 to 20 ounces peeled jicama, cut into ¼-inch-thick batons (I used
    2 9.5-ounce containers of precut jicama sticks from Trader Joe's)
1 tablespoon avocado oil

½ teaspoon garlic powder
¼ teaspoon chili powder (optional)
Freshly ground black pepper
Olive oil cooking spray

1. Make the herbed mayo: In a small, unheated skillet, combine the olive oil and garlic. Cook over low heat until the mixture begins to sizzle. Allow it to sizzle for 30 seconds, then transfer to a medium bowl. Let cool. Add the mayonnaise, lemon zest and juice, parsley, and dill to the bowl; fold until well combined. (Alternatively, you can blend the ingredients in the bowl of a small food processor until smooth.) Taste and season with salt and pepper. (This will yield about ⅔ cup.)
2. Make the fries: Bring a saucepan of salted water to a boil. Add the jicama, bring back to a boil, and boil for 10 minutes. Drain; pat the jicama dry thoroughly.
3. Preheat an air fryer to 400°F.
4. Toss the jicama with the avocado oil, garlic powder, and chili powder. Season with pepper. Mist the air fryer basket with cooking spray. Place the fries in the basket in a single layer. (Do not overcrowd the fryer; work in batches, if needed.) Air fry for 18 to 20 minutes, until the fries are golden and crisp, shaking the basket halfway through. Serve the fries hot, with the herbed mayo.

PER SERVING (A QUARTER OF THE FRIES WITH 2 TABLESPOONS MAYO): 318 calories, 1g protein, 31g fat, 13g carbohydrates, 7g fiber

NOTES:

You can make the mayo up to 1 day ahead; keep covered in the fridge. If you have extra, stir it into canned tuna or salmon.

If you're making the fries in batches, keep the first ones warm in the oven. Set your oven to 200°F and line a baking sheet with a wire rack misted with cooking spray. Place the cooked fries on the rack in the oven while you cook the remaining fries.

Romesco Dip

This luscious, tangy dip is my version of the Spanish sauce made with roasted peppers and almonds. It's delicious right out of the processor, but even better if it sits for a day, so make it in advance if you have the time. Serve it with vegetables for dunking, slather it on grain-free crackers— you can even spread it on a burger or a piece of grilled chicken or fish.

PREP: 15 minutes
COOK: 2 minutes
YIELD: 1¼ cups

> 2 tablespoons extra-virgin olive oil
> 3 garlic cloves, minced (1 tablespoon)
> 1 cup drained jarred roasted red peppers
> ⅓ cup smooth unsweetened almond butter
> 1 tablespoon chopped fresh flat-leaf parsley
> 2 teaspoons red wine vinegar
> ½ teaspoon hot paprika
> Pinch of cayenne (optional)
> ¼ teaspoon raw honey
> Fine sea salt and freshly ground black pepper

1. Combine the olive oil and garlic in a small, unheated skillet over low heat. Cook until the mixture begins to sizzle. Allow it to sizzle for 1 minute, then transfer to a small bowl to cool.
2. In the bowl of a food processor, combine the roasted peppers, almond butter, parsley, vinegar, paprika, cayenne if using, and honey. Add the cooled garlic mixture. Blend until smooth, stopping to scrape down the sides and bottom of the bowl. Taste and season with salt and pepper.
3. Serve, or cover and refrigerate to serve later.

PER SERVING (2 TABLESPOONS): 84 calories, 2g protein, 7g fat, 5g carbohydrates, 1g fiber

Appendix

. . . .

Best Practices and Resources

Electrolytes

https://www.cynthiathurlow.com/

Simply Hydration is an exciting electrolyte blend designed specifically for health- and performance-oriented individuals. Each 3 mL serving provides 75 mg magnesium and 300 mg chloride sourced from ionic trace minerals, 150 mg sodium (from seawater), and 150 mg potassium (as potassium chloride). Ionic minerals are readily absorbed, which allows for rapid replenishment.

This concentrated formula is convenient for adding to water or other beverages and can be used by individuals who may benefit from increased electrolyte intake while intermittent fasting.

MCT Oil

https://www.cynthiathurlow.com/

Simply Energy is 100 percent pure caprylic acid sourced exclusively from coconut oil. Each 1-tablespoon serving provides 14 grams of caprylic acid convenient for adding to coffee or tea, using in shakes and smoothies, or incorporating into recipes as needed. Caprylic acid is a medium-chain fatty acid with 8 carbon atoms, hence its chemical shorthand, C8. Medium-chain fatty acids have unique properties that distinguish them from other fatty acids by giving them the utility for adding to ketogenic diets and for incorporating them into other dietary approaches.

Resistant Starch

https://www.cynthiathurlow.com/

Simply Fiber contains two forms of resistant starch (RS) type II: organic green banana flour and organic potato starch powder. RS is a type of starch that is resistant to digestion, as enzymes in the gastrointestinal (GI) tract are inactive against it. Once RS reaches the large intestine, it is fermented into short-chain fatty acids, which are used as fuel for both beneficial microbes and enterocytes of the GI tract. Simply Fiber benefits GI health through its ability to support microbial balance and proper intestinal permeability and integrity. Additionally, this formula may help support optimal blood sugar and insulin metabolism, normal appetite, and cardiovascular health.

Protein Powder

https://www.cynthiathurlow.com/
Simply Protein is a novel, great-tasting, dairy-free protein powder, yielding 21 grams of protein per serving. It contains HydroBEEF™, a highly concentrated, bone broth protein isolate, produced through an exclusive proprietary process that allows the protein to be hydrolyzed into more peptides, resulting in easier absorption and assimilation. This product contains beef from animals raised in Sweden without hormones or antibiotics and is free of any GMO grains, grasses, and/or ensilage.

HCL

https://shop.bioticsresearch.com/
https://klaire.com/
Hydro-Zyme by Biotics Research or Klaire Labs

Digestive Enzymes

https://enzymedica.com/
https://www.thorne.com/
Digest Spectrum by Enzymedica or Bio-Gest by Thorne Labs

Healthy Juice

https://theweeklyjuicery.lpages.co/cynthia-thurlow-guided-juice-fast/
Are you ready to Chase Good Health and feel AMAZING? This Guided One-Day Juice Fast with The Weekly Juicery floods our body with organic plants, provides much needed digestive rest time, and helps reset our sugar barometer so we crave more fruits and vegetables!

Glucose Monitor & App

https://nutrisense.io

Face Cleanser

https://www.tataharperskincare.com/

Eye Cream
https://www.beautycounter.com/cynthiathurlow
BeautyCounter Countermatch

GI Detox
https://biocidin.com/products/gi-detox

Spermidine
https://spermidinelife.us/

Berberine
https://shop.designsforhealth.com/

Dihydroberberine
https://nnbnutrition.com/products/glucovantage/
Glucovantage by NNB

Chromium GTF
https://www.orthomolecularproducts.com/

Medicinal Mushrooms
https://us.foursigmatic.com/

Adaptogenic Herbs
Piquetea.com
Ashwagandha, Rhodiola, Maca

Apple Cider Vinegar
https://www.bragg.com/
Bragg's with Mother

Acknowledgments

After I left clinical medicine five years ago and devoted my experience and expertise to intermittent fasting and female health, I had no idea that one day I would write a book on this critically important topic. Yet here it is—and the writing of this book has been a remarkable, yet humbling experience, especially among a global pandemic, social distancing, and two teens schooling at home throughout the process. Along the way I learned that the creation of a book is very much a team collaboration, in which many people play huge, diverse, and vitally important roles. I have so many people to thank for supporting me, educating me, and helping me bring this dream and project to fruition.

To Chris Winfield, who was instrumental in connecting me with my literary agent, Anna Petkovich at Park Fine. Anna, thank you for believing in me, guiding me through the process of creating the basic blueprint of this book, being a sounding board when I needed one, and helping me navigate finding the perfect publisher to bring this book and ideas to so many.

To my literary team at Penguin Random House, Lucia Watson and Suzy Swartz—who are absolutely remarkable and insightful at what they do. After I met them, I knew I had the best editing team in the business. Thank you for your support throughout this process!

To JJ Virgin, for your insight, business acumen, and inspiration, which spurred me to greater achievements . . . and RISING to the occasion.

To JJ Virgin and Karl Krummenacher and my entire Mindshare Mastermind community . . . thank you for all the love, encouragement, and support. Truly the most heart-centered entrepreneurs I know.

To Jaime Pallotolo, my mindset guru and friend, thank you for seeing the potential in me before I did, and for all your love and support.

To Teri Cochrane, your mentorship, friendship, and energetic potential is boundless. There are zero coincidences, and I'm so glad you are in my life.

To Tucker Stine, for your enthusiasm, positivity, and endless professional narratives. One talk really can change your life. I appreciate your investment in my vision and commitment to seeing this all through fresh eyes.

To Tony Whatley, thank you for pushing me to not play SMALL, especially in 2019. Carpe diem!

To my team and IF:45 coaches at www.cynthiathurlow.com, who are so hardworking, professional, dedicated, and truly special. Thank you.

To Beth Lipton, definitely one of the BEST chefs in the country, with an extraordinary ability to develop recipes and meals that are not only nutrient dense, but delicious beyond belief. Beth, you are a culinary rock star!

To Maggie Greenwood-Robinson, who really understood what I wanted to convey in words and helped me achieve it by organizing the material into a wonderful flow and did so under a very tight deadline . . . while encouraging me to focus on the big picture and not get caught up in the pace and stress of writing. Thank you for keeping me calm, level-headed, and on track.

To my parents, thank you for instilling in me a stubborn tenaciousness and love for learning; to my brother, thank you for always forcing me to laugh at myself and not take life too seriously.

To my extended family and close friends . . . thank you for allowing me to share this experience with you, and for your love and support. Without it, I would not be who I am today.

And to those colleagues who, unknowingly, inspired me to pursue and embrace fasting and metabolic health, including Dr. Jason Fung; Dr Gabrielle Lyon; Dr Ben Bikman; Dr Peter Attia; Dr Ken Berry; Dr David Jockers; Dr. Brian Lenzkes; Dr Daniel Pompa; Dr. Tro Kalayjian; Dr Cate Shanahan; Dr. Mindy Pelz; Dave Asprey; Siim Land; Ben Azadi; Robb Wolfe; Jimmy Moore; Marty Kendall; Shawn Wells; Melanie Avalon; Gin Stephens; Megan Ramos; Maria Emmerich; and female hormonal health experts Dr. Sara Gottfried, Dr. Anna Cabeca, Dr. Carrie Jones, Dr. Lisa Mosconi, Dr. Jaime Seeman, and so many more. I appreciate your contributions to my growing knowledge base and the impact it makes in so many lives!

And, lastly, to my appendix . . . I never appreciated you until you ruptured, but my thirteen-day hospitalization is what got this entire journey accelerated. Feeling compelled and called to do my second TEDx Talk is what started the second half of my journey, and I'm grateful for the journey.

Index

Note: *Italicized* page numbers indicate material in tables or illustrations.